To Do No Harm

To Do No Harm

DES and the Dilemmas
of Modern Medicine

Roberta J. Apfel, M.D., M. P. H.
Susan M. Fisher, M.D.

Yale University Press
New Haven and London

Published with assistance from the foundation established in memory of Philip Hamilton McMillan of the Class of 1894, Yale College.

Designed by Nancy Ovedovitz and set in VIP Baskerville type by The Composing Room of Mich., Inc. Printed in the United States of America by Murray Printing Company, Westford, Massachusetts.

Library of Congress Cataloging in Publication Data

Apfel, Roberta J., 1938–
    To do no harm.
    Bibliography: p.
    Includes index.
    1. Diethylstilbestrol—Toxicology. 2. Vagina—Cancer—Psychological aspects. 3. Physician and patient. 4. Trust (Psychology) 5. Iatrogenic diseases—Psychological aspects. I. Fisher, Susan M., 1937– II. Title. [DNLM:
    1. Diethylstilbestrol—Adverse effects.
    2. Diethylstilbestrol—History. 3. Prenatal exposure delayed effects. 4. Physician-patient relations. WP522 A641t]
    RA1242.D48A64 1984   363.1'94   84–5089

ISBN 0–300–03192–0

The paper in this book meets the guidelines for permanence and durability of the Committee on Production Guidelines for Book Longevity of the Council on Library Resources.

10   9   8   7   6   5   4   3   2

For Bennett and Herman

He has not claimed to be wise or asserted
that wisdom is possible; he has only
argued that through discourse
philosophy, the search for wisdom, is
viable.
　　　　　　—Herman Sinaiko,
Love, Knowledge, and Discourse in Plato

Contents

Preface

This book began with a conversation between us on the cliffs at Ogunquit, Maine. Its present form has emerged from three years of further conversation with each other and with family, colleagues, patients, and friends both old and new—all of whom shared in some measure our interests and our concern and each of whom made a special contribution to our efforts.

To those of our professional colleagues who have been active participants in the story of DES, our special thanks for the generosity with which they shared their hard-gained knowledge with us in many hours of conversation: Ann Barnes, Susan Bell, Marluce Bibbo, Louis Burke, Ralph Engle, Elaine Gutterman, Alice Hamm, Arthur Herbst, Herbert Horne, Jr., Marion Hubby, Lorna Johnson, Richard Pillard, Stanley Robboy, Samuel Shapiro, Olive Smith, and Gail Strassfield.

As the work progressed, our ideas were constantly expanded and tested by the thoughtful criticism of many friends and acquaintances. We are particularly grateful for our discussions and correspondence with Polly Apfel, Judith Barnard, Joel Beck, Rhonda Blair, Margaret Brenman-Gibson, Iain Chalmers, Michael Fain, John Grover, Judith Lumley, Leah Mason-Beck, Susan Noakes, Celia Savitz, Kathleen Rudd Scharf, William Schultz, Sandra Siler, William Silverman, John Simms, and Jeanne Springer.

We owe a special debt to Jeffrey Scott Stern. In his painstaking editing of the manuscript he shared with us his splendid appreciation of literary style and of psychoanalysis.

At various stages of the project we called upon many individuals in diverse fields for assistance in research. Our deep thanks for such help goes to Kalman Apfel, Robert Binstock, Andrea Goldstein, Martha Izzi, Marvin Leon, Molly Savitz, Betty Wechter, Dacia Wolfson, and Beth Zimmerman.

The Rockefeller Foundation awarded a residential scholarship at Bellagio, Italy, which supported work on this book.

Gladys Topkis, with her humor, tact, and warmth, has made the experience of being edited a pleasure.

And finally, for those private debts of inspiration and love which can never be repaid but require some public acknowledgment, our thanks to Emma Goldman, Charles Magraw, and Jacob Swartz; to our children, Amy, Benjamin, Celia, Debby, Jonathan, Michael, and Molly; and, above all, to our husbands, Bennett Simon and Herman Sinaiko.

To Do No Harm

Introduction

If my history be judged useful by those inquirers who desire an exact knowledge of the past as an aid to the interpretation of the future, which in the course of human things must resemble if it does not reflect it, I shall be content.
   —Thucydides, *The Peloponnesian War*

Diethylstilbestrol (DES) is a synthetic estrogen first produced in 1938. It has since been used for a wide variety of medical conditions, including prevention of pregnancy complications from the 1940's until 1971 when the Food and Drug Administration (FDA) required product labeling to state that DES was contraindicated for use in the prevention of miscarriages. It is estimated that 4 to 6 million Americans (mothers, daughters, and sons) were exposed to DES during pregnancy. Although DES is a synthetic estrogen and differs in structure and metabolism from naturally occurring estrogens, many investigators believe that there is no evidence that natural and synthetic estrogen differ in biologic effect (including toxic effects).

Studies have shown a clear association between the occurrence of a rare form of malignant vaginal cancer, clear cell adenocarcinoma, with intrauterine exposure to DES. In addition, many DES daughters were found to have a benign vaginal condition called adenosis. This condition is characterized by the presence of non-malignant glandular tissue in the vagina.

1

More recently, a follow-up study at the University of Chicago revealed more breast and gynecological cancers among exposed mothers than among a control group, although the difference was not statistically significant. A follow-up of DES mothers at the Mayo Clinic did not reveal any increases, but the dose of DES was on the average lower in the Mayo Clinic group.

In addition, recent studies have shown an excess of abnormalities in the genital and possibly lower urinary tract in DES-exposed males. A DES Task Force was formed in February by the Office of the Assistant Secretary for Health to examine the health effects of DES in pregnancy. The group examined the current state of medical knowledge concerning the drug's effects and made recommendations for immediate action as well as future research. This Advisory outlines the Task Force's recommendations to assist you in managing your patients who may have had pregnancy exposure to DES. (Richmond 1978)

This advisory letter, with its flat, matter-of-fact tone about a medical disaster, was mailed to all licensed physicians in the United States in October 1978. By the time we received this official warning, seven years had elapsed since the FDA ruling that DES was "contraindicated for use in the prevention of miscarriages." During this period both of us had already been touched by the DES tragedy. We had seen DES-related anxieties and physical conditions in family, friends, and colleagues. Since 1978, the consequences have mounted. Insidiously and ironically, infertility has been added to the possible effects of DES on male and female offspring: the drug given to enhance reproduction did not do so, and that same drug has now inhibited reproduction in a second generation.

We decided to collaborate on this book in 1980—after the initial wave of turmoil and publicity about DES had faded and when "all-clear" signals were being sounded (Elliott 1979, Knox 1980). We feared that the public would be lulled into thinking there was no longer any problem subsequent to DES use and that comfortable resolution had been achieved. We worried that individual vigilance might cease under premature reassurance from professional experts. We believe that there are continuing, if more subtle, problems which are direct consequences of DES, problems that merit fuller discussion and understanding.

Beyond these concerns, we see DES as a paradigm of the peculiarly modern phenomenon in which large-scale destructive consequences of a medical or technological innovation emerge unexpectedly as much as a generation after a benign or inconsequential beginning. A second, even more far-reaching aspect of the DES story is that it encapsulates in a quite remarkable fashion the whole complex history and structure of modern medicine in relation to modern life.

In some respects, the DES story is a twentieth-century medical detective story. Yet the facts have been public and well known for over a decade, and the villains are absent or obscure. More important, the whole episode could happen again at any time.

As psychiatrists, we were initially impressed with what we know best—the emotional effects of DES on the patients we see in our clinical practices. Our interest has extended from the intrapersonal and interpersonal spheres in two directions: to the larger social and psychological arenas in which the DES story and others like it are played out and to the biological level, where the interaction of substances such as DES with the human body may be examined.

We first explore the history of DES in relation to the social setting, to the general history of medicine, and to the emerging scientific research establishment. It is an extremely complex and multidimensional story, involving the relation between mother and child, the relation between patient and doctor—in this instance the woman and her gynecologist, the relation between doctors and their peers, and the relation of the medical community to the larger society. We look not only at overt dimensions of these relationships but also at aspects that are not apparent to the participants. We feel that this unconscious dimension, to which we as psychiatrists and psychoanalysts are especially sensitive, is both the most problematic and the most significant facet, and that without it the story remains largely unintelligible and fragmentary.

The passions engendered through the entire history of DES are such as to make objective understanding nearly impossible. Almost automatically, writers on the subject fall into partisan postures. One group, unremittingly hostile to the medical profession, views DES mothers and their offspring simply as innocent victims for whom outraged and righteous indignation is the only possible response. Other writers defend medical practice by marshalling facts and figures and interpreting data in such a way as effectively to deny the significance of the entire event. The reasonable middle ground is rarely reflected in the existing literature.

Of course, we ourselves are not detached observers. Trained in American medicine, we are part of the system. In our work with patients, students, colleagues, and institutions, we struggle with the same problems the DES situation exemplifies. We believe that critiquing existing practice and theory is an important and valued tradition within medicine, though it is often ambivalently regarded.

Our overriding objective is to understand what happened, how it happened, what is happening and will continue to happen for all parties involved—and for society at large. We want to understand because we fear that ignorance of such a history must lead inevitably to its repetition.

Because the whole tangled history of DES is so intensely human, our comprehension of these events must be correspondingly humane. This means that the conventionally "objective" and emotionally abstract quality of science is not sufficient to our subject. But neither are moral outrage and indignation. It is here that our psychiatric background seems most relevant, for it provides us with a perspective from which to view these phenomena openly and without the wish merely to assess blame.

In addition to individual phenomena, we hope to illuminate institutional and cultural factors. The individuals with whom we are concerned, doctors and patients, interact with each other in socially and culturally prescribed roles. DES disrupted and disrupts these conventional roles, disturbing not only the individuals but also the cultural patterns and social processes within which they function. These social processes involve health policy makers, government regulatory agencies, and drug companies. Therefore we shall explore the DES story in its expanded dimensions as well.

When we began this project, we intended to study only the particular traumas engendered by DES. These include the complicated disillusionment that accompanies every large-scale public health disaster, but in the DES case these feelings are organized essentially around the disruption of the most private meanings of childbirth, bodily integrity, and deeply intimate human relationships.

As our work progressed, we observed the reluctance of the medical profession to implement requests for case-finding and follow-up by professional organizations and the Public Health Service Task Force. We became intrigued by the social and psychological context of a physician's life, training, and peer relationships, and by the internal regulatory mechanisms of the profession as well as by the complex character of physician-patient relationships.

At every turn, the study of DES reveals paradox and provokes surprise. There is, of course, an age-old conflict between the desire of the medical profession and the general public for bold new advances and the conservative conviction that the art of medicine works best when it helps nature to take its course—a conviction embodied in the writings of Hippocrates: *primum non nocere* (first of all, do no harm). But the contemporary arena in which this ancient struggle is played out has some novel features. Primary among them is the unprecedented rate of medical advance in this century, with attendant leaps in the human stakes involved.

So we tell a complicated, multifaceted, and multidisciplinary story whose meaning needs to be teased out from a welter of scientific facts, medical pronouncements, and ideological broadsides. There is no simple moral. Rather, the entire event needs to be seen in depth by a thoughtful and concerned public.

From the very beginning of our explorations, we were struck

by the fact that the emotional impact of DES had received almost no attention, although there have been continuous study and surveillance of its physical consequences. We initially became interested in DES when we saw young women in our analytic psychotherapy practices who happened to be DES daughters. These women did not come to therapy because of DES, but we felt that their DES exposure had had a profound and far-reaching effect upon them. Their interpretations of the DES experience had become a lens through which they viewed their relations with us, their doctors, as well as with their mothers, their boyfriends, lovers, husbands, and children. Their feelings and fantasies about DES were connected to their sense of their own conception and prenatal experience and to their future as mothers. Their bodily concerns were serious, continual, and realistic.

Then, as now, Dr. Louis Burke was seeing DES daughters in a colposcopy clinic at the Beth Israel Hospital in Boston. When she was a resident in psychiatry there, Dr. Johanna Gardner Shaw had interviewed some of the young women patients and was stunned by the frightening fantasies they shared with her about what DES had done to their bodies. Many women do not know what their internal organs look like. This lack of knowledge and the realistic fear of organ damage or abnormality can produce bizarre fantasies. In the case of DES daughters, the knowledge that things were somehow awry stimulated horrific visions. On the basis of preliminary interviews, Dr. Burke introduced a video machine into the clinic by means of which patients could see their own organs and the adenosis and other structural changes due to DES. This experience apparently relieved much of their anxiety. However, Dr. Burke, an unusually sensitive gynecologist, wondered whether something else might be offered, such as a discussion group. He therefore asked us to talk with the daughters and their mothers to assess their emotional stress and help determine how to deal with it. At the same time, the local chapter of DES Action, a national group of DES mothers and daughters, was running leaderless discussion groups and wanted professional advice. They had contacted Dr. Burke and asked him to help establish a congenial setting in which the emotional concerns of their members could be addressed along with physical ones. He passed this responsibility on to us.[1]

Thus, at the time we were becoming increasingly interested in DES, Dr. Burke's invitation and referral provided opportunities to learn and do more about it. In the course of a little more than a year, we met individually with fifty daughters and mothers. We also met with a group of ten mothers and daughters to discuss what DES meant to them. We read several hundred letters that were received by DES Action from DES-exposed persons who were seeking advice or commenting on their personal agonies. We have presented some of our findings since 1977 in "Psychological Impact of Diethylstilbestrol Exposure *in Utero*," an article written for practicing gynecologists (Burke et al. 1980). We have also given papers at national and local meetings of psychiatrists, psychoanalysts, medical students, public health students, medical faculties, and obstetricians and gynecologists. These settings have provided further opportunities to broaden our understanding of the emotional consequences of DES. Our interest has led to consultations with community agencies and colleagues, and with DES-connected individuals of all ages. We interviewed three mothers involved in a lawsuit prior to trial and reviewed testimony of ten other litigants who had been subjects in studies conducted between 1950 and 1952 at the Chicago Lying-In Hospital (Mink et al. 1982). All told, we have seen or heard about several hundred situations.

We recognize, of course, that we have seen a biased sample comprised of those who have sought us out for help or counsel, if only for a quick chat after a lecture. We do not know for certain whether the effects we have observed and described are *absolutely* causally related to DES in every instance. Yet some psychological findings that we associate with DES appear to be different from what we find in other patients we treat and people we meet. We think this is significant. Carefully controlled studies based on specific hypotheses that compare DES-exposed and nonexposed populations are needed in the behavioral area as in drug research. Such hypotheses, however, can originate only out of clinical descriptions and in-depth interviews such as those we present. A few people, notably Anke Ehrhardt and Heino Meyer-Bahlburg, have begun controlled studies which attempt to distinguish the effects of DES per se from those of other factors, such as the fear of any cancer.[2]

We seek to understand the DES experience within the framework of other significant emotional experiences. We are interested in the ways in which stress related to DES resembles and differs from other kinds of stress. Finally, we seek to understand the havoc a drug can wreak on the soul and psyche as well as on the human body.

There is one other phenomenon that arose from our dealings with DES mothers and daughters and led directly to our writing this book. After we began to report our findings about DES to various audiences, we gradually became aware of a peculiar response: no matter whom we addressed—medical researchers, practicing physicians, DES mothers and daughters, academics, or laypersons—and no matter what the form of our talk—public panel discussions, hospital grand rounds, private counseling sessions, even dinner-table and cocktail-party conversations—the people to whom we described our findings always failed to grasp what we were saying at first. They wanted to know who was responsible for the disaster—who profited by it, either in money or reputation or public honors. They wanted to know who had deceived the public and why. They wanted, in short, the secret, inside story of how the scandal occurred. We had to tell them that there was no inside story, no significant heroes and villains; that the scandal is intrinsic to the very structure of modern medicine.

It took us some time to grasp why our audience always initially misunderstood our story. The cause, we now think, is twofold. On the one hand the events we described did not fit the conventional pattern of historical narratives because the behavior of the actors and their conscious motivations do not account for what happened. On the other hand, the more complex, less conventional account that we believe to be the truer one produced a sense of helplessness and anxiety in our audience. If there are no villains, what are the remedies?

Of course we believe that mistakes were made, that procedures were not adequate, and that the range of available scientific research resources was not fully utilized. But it is not clear how much difference any of this made—or how much difference the technical improvements of recent decades will make the next time around. (It should go without saying that no one could have anticipated the disastrous long-term consequences of taking DES.)

We want not only to tell the story but to overcome public resistance to hearing it and confronting its implications. The major significance of the DES tale for us lies in the clarity with which it exposes deep, fundamental, and often difficult-to-perceive aspects of modern medicine. If our account seems to wander through some strange byways—psychoanalytic theory, the history of medicine, the dynamics of medical education—we beg the reader's indulgence; for these are not digressions but essential aspects of the story we are trying to tell.

1

The History of DES

It is difficult to call to mind any subject upon which
more rubbish has been written than the sex hormones.
This is very largely the result of the general public's
desire for the maintenance of youth and all that it
implies, together with the successful exploitation of
this trait by commercial firms.
    —Charles Dodds, 1934

Five years after making this remark, Dodds was knighted for his
key role in the synthesis of sex hormones.

The middle years of the twentieth century saw an explosion of
medical research, new drug therapies, and advances in medical
technology. An America that could win great wars, create nuclear
arms, and send rockets into space surely could attack the everyday problems of personal health. There was a renewed belief in
medicine as a source of answers to the basic questions and yearnings of mankind. It was a time of optimism about conquering
human ills. Medical warfare could be waged against high infant
mortality, and premature babies would be saved. The problems
of sexuality and reproduction would be mastered.

The DES story touches on every element of medical culture in
the past five decades. It also replicates earlier historical patterns.
In its development and usage, DES recalls many other medical
discoveries that have enjoyed brief popularity and then lost favor.

Yet DES is also unique to the twentieth century and its dramatic increases in material wealth and complex technology. DES was one of many treatments that were rapidly adopted but ultimately may have resulted in greater harm than the conditions they were designed to relieve.

DES is a man-made, or synthetic, hormone, and hormones have become the focus of intense medical attention and research in this century. Natural hormones are substances secreted in one part of an animal's body that act upon organ systems elsewhere in the body, promoting growth and regulating a variety of complex functions. Synthetic hormones are substances made in a laboratory that simulate the effects of the naturally occurring hormones. Before 1900, there were no techniques to demonstrate the structure and function of hormones; their existence was only theoretical. Enormous effort went into discovering the nature of hormones. The excitement underlying the new specialty of endocrinology was rooted in the fascination with prolonging youth and the wish to master the secrets of sexuality and fertility.

The ovaries release eggs and produce two female sex hormones, progesterone and estrogen, which influence the reproductive cycle. In most mammals, estrogen produces *estrus*, a period of sexual excitement during which conception can occur. The word comes from the Greek *oistros*, meaning gadfly, sting, or frenzy; from that comes the further meaning "strong impulse and overwhelming desire." The word *hormone* comes from the Greek *hormān*, to spur on or set in motion. In human females, however, estrogens act to build the lining of the uterus, which will later be shed during menstruation if fertilization has not taken place; sexual excitation is not linked directly to the production of estrogen hormone.

The ancient Greeks recognized the effects of estrogen, but it was not until 1912 that biologically active extracts of ovaries were discovered. In 1923 a biological assay was developed to measure the capacity of a hormone to induce estrus in laboratory animals.[1] By 1927, Selmar Aschheim and Bernhardt Zondek had demonstrated that the urine of pregnant animals contained excessive oestrin which caused estrus in immature mice, the basis of the first pregnancy test.[2] In 1929, Edward Doisy and his co-workers in England, and Adolph Butenandt in Germany, both isolated nearly pure, natural estrogenic compounds. These were very popular, but also very costly and difficult to produce. Natural estrogens derived from the urine of pregnant horses and pigs were purified for use in experimental animals and in human patients. They had to be given by painful injection and often caused abscesses. High cost restricted their use to wealthy patients. In 1932 Charles Dodds wrote that oestrin had been seriously recommended for all types of menstrual disorders, for every form of insanity, for the treatment of vascular disease in men, and for hemophilia. He noted that sex hormones were so popular that it was only the difficulty of obtaining them that prevented their use in every condition from simple hives to megalomania. He made a plea for carefully controlled observations and selective use of estrogens for menstrual and menopausal problems.

Patients, doctors, researchers, and drug companies all wanted a cheap, easily produced, standard form of synthetic estrogen. Then, in 1938, Dodds and his co-workers sent a letter to the editor of *Nature* announcing the syntheses of oestrogenic substances. Colleagues at the Courtauld Institute in London and at Oxford had collaborated to produce what they called the "mother substance"—stilbestrol, and related compounds. Diethylstilbestrol (DES) was a relatively simple structure (see figure, chapter 3) easily manufactured from coal tar. It produced effects identical to the natural substance. Other synthetic estrogens followed, and eventually about one hundred brands were introduced.[3]

DES immediately became a tremendous success. It was more potent than the natural estrogen, requiring far less than the biological extract to produce the same effect. It could be produced cheaply and in pure form, and it could be administered by mouth. And because DES was discovered under a grant from the British Medical Research Council, whose policy it was that new discoveries should be well publicized and not patented, DES became widely available very quickly. Its inexpensiveness appealed to the drug industry, and its purity attracted the investigative scientists, as did the fact that milligram for milligram it was more powerful than natural estrogens.

By the time Dodds gave the Cameron Prize lecture in 1941, he had become as enthusiastic about the clinical uses of DES as he had previously been cautious about natural estrogens. DES, he said, heralded "a new era." By 1939 it was already popular in the United Kingdom, France, Germany, Sweden, and the United States, where it was used to treat menopausal complaints, amenorrhea, and genital underdevelopment, and to suppress lactation. One indication of the extraordinary popularity of DES is that in the three years after its synthesis, 257 papers—an enormous number for any subject—appeared in the medical and scientific literature describing various animal experiments with the drug and clinical uses for it (Noller and Fish 1974).

As compared to natural estrogen, DES was in every way more effective—and more toxic. Carcinogenic potency is proportional to estrogenic activity, and estrogens had been implicated by Loeb in the development of tumors as early as 1919. In 1936 Loeb's group showed that natural estrogen produces carcinoma-like proliferation of the vagina, cervix, and uterus in mice. Mammary-gland tumors, which occur with high frequency in mice, can be more rapidly induced by estrogenic substances, and in 1939, the same year that DES was synthesized, it was reported that stilbestrol injections had expedited the development of breast cancer in two mice. In the following year, a mammary carcinoma in a rat was reported. A 1940 study from the National Institutes of Health compared the carcinogenic potency of synthetic and natural estrogen and concluded that both types "showed toxic manifestations only in genital and breast tissues."[4]

In the early 1940s commercial agricultural use of DES began. From the end of World War II, DES-supplemented feed was given to livestock and chickens. Farmers decreased their feeding costs by using DES because the animals achieved a higher weight in a shorter time period. DES produced marbling in red meat and juicier chickens, thus increasing their market value. The FDA banned the use of DES pellets for chickens and lambs in 1959, when high DES levels in meat were discovered to produce distressing symptoms in consumers.[5] From 1969 on, the FDA and cattle breeders struggled over regulations to prohibit DES in cattle feed.[6] In 1979, the Department of Agriculture finally prohibited the supplementation of animal feed with DES, but scattered reports indicate that it continues to be used covertly today.[7]

DES was approved for medical use in human beings in September 1941. Its approval is intertwined with the development of drug regulation in twentieth-century America. Sociologist Susan Bell's dissertation, "The Synthetic Compound Diethylstilbestrol (DES) 1938–1941: The Social Construction of a Medical Treatment" (1980), superbly details the political and social complexities of this time period and is our source for the following summary of DES licensure.

The federal government established the Bureau of Chemistry in the nineteenth century to control adulterated food, and in 1906 the Food and Drug Act was passed to regulate and research drugs and food. The 1906 act defined drugs broadly as substances intended to cure, mitigate, or prevent disease. Proprietary, or patent, medicines (commercially produced and available without a physician's prescription) were particularly affected by the new law. The manufacturers of prescription, or "ethical," drugs, such as Lilly, Abbott, Squibb, Upjohn, and Parke-Davis, only started to expand in the 1920s. Until then, most physicians concocted medicines for individual patients or recommended patent medicines. In the 1930s drug companies moved to further distinguish their ethical products from proprietary substances; they began to relate to the regulatory agency and to advise the government about drugs.[8]

In 1923, Walter G. Campbell became acting chief of the Bureau of Chemistry; he focused further critical attention on drug regulation and, at the same time, began a policy of cooperation with the prescription drug manufacturers. In 1927, a new agency, the Food, Drug and Insecticide Administration, was established within the Department of Agriculture to do the regulatory work and research necessary for enforcement of the 1906 act. In

1930, its name was changed to the Food and Drug Administration (FDA). Campbell became commissioner of the FDA, a post he retained until 1944.

By the mid-1930s, Campbell and other FDA officials began to seek support from Congress and the public for passage of a new act that would further regulate the food, drug, and cosmetic market. The early 1930s saw considerable activism from national women's organizations, Consumers' Research, and other consumer groups that favored more government regulation of business.

The New Deal was characterized by its volatile public discussion of social issues. The drug law that would replace the 1906 act was passionately debated from its introduction in 1933 until its passage in 1938 as the Food, Drug, and Cosmetic Act. The consumer support essential for its passage was not sufficient to carry it through for five years. Ethical (i.e., prescription) drug companies originally opposed the bill; after five years of debate and revision, these companies had either come to support it or had dropped their opposition to it. The FDA responded to the increased demands placed on it by the 1938 act by establishing the New Drugs Division. The newly reorganized agency was woefully underfunded by Congress in the period 1938–41, when it was being flooded by an average of one hundred new drug applications per month. During this process, the drug industry allied itself with the medical profession and disavowed any connection with patent medicines. Most of the reforms enacted in 1938 were aimed at proprietary, not ethical, substances. The key concept in this reform was the requirement for safety.

DES was the first important medicinal substance to be considered under the 1938 act in light of this new requirement. The highest standards in U.S. history were applied to consideration of DES. The DES application was a challenge to the FDA's ability to protect the public and at the same time supply important new medicines expeditiously.

"Safety" is a relative concept. It is not specifically defined by law. For a "life-saving" drug such as sulfa, already approved, the safety criteria did not have to be as stringent as for DES because without intervention the illnesses sulfa was used to treat would lead to death. By contrast, DES was proposed as a "life-enhancing" drug; hence considerations of side effects were more complex. When saving a life is at issue, many more discomforts are tolerated than when the focus is merely on improving the quality of life.[9]

The review of DES was extensive. Each manufacturer had to file a New Drug Application (NDA) for each preparation and dosage. FDA chemists, medical officers, and pharmacologists then reviewed published and unpublished reports of studies on DES. The FDA commissioner, Walter G. Campbell, the Drugs Division chief, Theodore G. Klumpp, and the New Drugs Division chief, J. J. Durrett, were all involved in the data review and in personal interviews with physicians, researchers, and academic scientists through 1939 and 1940. The entire FDA medical staff participated in the review of DES data. Klumpp has since testified that they met almost daily to discuss events.

The first NDAs submitted by individual drug manufacturers were rejected or withdrawn in 1939 because they were judged to be incomplete and demonstrated insufficient proof of safety. The FDA then decided to hear *en masse* from the companies that had applications on file in December 1940. Twelve companies produced a "Master File" in May 1941.[10] Representatives of these drug companies worked with the FDA staff to amass evidence from fifty-four experts representing academic centers across the nation. The agency saved time and money by encouraging such joint applications, by reviewing the NDAs informally, and by cooperating with professional friends and colleagues in the drug industry to whom reviews could be delegated. In addition, the FDA received 138 testimonial letters and about 5,000 case reports from clinicians who had used the drug. All but four of the fifty-four academic experts gave their approval to DES as a "safe" drug: Ephraim Shorr and his co-workers at Cornell Medical Center in 1939 had found DES toxic in their trials for amenorrhea (failure to menstruate); it produced severe nausea and vomiting in as many as 80 percent of the women.

The four doctors who held out against DES approval were seen as standing in the way of progress.[11] As a concession to them, DES was approved for limited usage where its safety seemed clearly established: to treat vaginitis, gonorrhea, and menopausal symptoms, and to suppress lactation. A warning was placed on the physician instruction sheet not to use the drug for amenorrhea.

Another early concern, which in hindsight seems prescient, was that the drug would be used too generally and inappropriately. Once FDA approval was granted, the drug could be used by unsupervised physicians for any reason. There was no way to prevent this. Usage did generalize quickly and was extended to the treatment of amenorrhea, dysmenorrhea (painful or difficult menses), pregnancy problems including nausea and vomiting, infertility, toxemia, diabetes, and other high-risk medical conditions. Drug salesmen, known as "detail men," suggested these expanded uses of DES to physicians in private practice. Low dosage was suggested by the FDA, and contraindications for usage were issued based on the known risks from all estrogens—evidence of cancerous or precancerous lesions of the breast or cervix or a family history of breast or genital cancer. But the information given to both the general public and the general physician was incomplete. This was seen by the FDA as a way of protecting the consumer. The patient had to go to a physician, who would prescribe and explain the medicine to the best of his or her knowledge. In contrast, self-medication with patent or proprietary remedies was considered to be of lowest quality. General medical care such as this was thought to be of intermediate quality, and care by an academic specialist was considered to be the highest quality.

The government felt that the safety criterion had been met. Clinicians, however, were also concerned about efficacy. The requirement to prove efficacy was not introduced until 1962. A drug that is effective may be used even when it is relatively unsafe if the benefits of the treatment are believed to outweigh its risks.

The dilemmas and questions that emerged around DES between 1938 and 1941 exemplify two major concerns about drug approval that continue to this day: the quality of research, and the frequently conflicting interests of consumers, physicians, drug companies, and government agencies. In 1939 an editorial in the *Journal of the American Medical Association* reflecting upon reports on stilbestrol warned against the indiscriminate and unscientific use of estrogens, specifically naming DES.[12] Nevertheless, there was great pressure on the FDA to approve DES from clinicians, sex researchers, the fledgling drug industry, and consumers eager to try sex hormones.

In retrospect, it appears that, given the groundswell of shared enthusiasm for DES, given the quality of drug evaluation in 1940, given the absence of efficacy as a criterion, and given the interdependence of the parties, there was no way the review of DES could have come out differently. The few skeptical critics with a historical perspective were not heeded. This historical example raises questions for our time. Despite our increasingly sophisticated knowledge of long-term side effects of drugs and the new focus on efficacy, are we any better protected from the same tendency toward consensus of public, academic, and commercial interests that existed with DES? Despite the new restraints, problematic drugs are still being licensed, drugs are still being used for purposes that are not officially sanctioned, and unanticipated, drastic effects still erupt.

The original clinical uses for which DES was approved in 1941 were to treat gonorrheal vaginitis, senile vaginitis, and menopausal symptoms, and to suppress lactation. Previously established medical uses of natural estrogen were continued with the new compound DES. In the treatment of men with cancer of the prostate, DES had already proved life-prolonging by suppressing the male hormone, testosterone, which stimulates tumor growth. (An unfortunate side effect of this use of DES is feminization of the male patient.) Of the original uses for women, the treatment of gonorrhea with DES was soon discontinued because it did not work and effective antibiotics became available. The use of DES to treat menopausal symptoms and to halt lactation continued.

It is noteworthy that DES was not initially approved for any usage whatever during pregnancy. Between 1941 and 1947, it was used during pregnancy without FDA approval (Karnaky 1942, Smith and Smith 1946). In 1947, partly in response to studies by Olive Smith and George Smith, several drug companies filed a supplementary NDA to permit the use of DES during pregnancy and to allow the production of a 25 mg pill in addition to the 1, 2, and 5 mg pills. This request was granted. In 1952, the FDA declared DES to be safe and no longer a new drug requiring annual approval. Stunningly, the expansion of DES usage to pregnancy and the introduction of larger doses were done by simple administrative fiat. No new research data or reviews were required, and the use of DES was now exempted from official regulatory constraint.[13]

Beyond sanctioning specific treatment uses for DES, the FDA approval cleared the way for more intensive research into other uses for this new drug. One center of sex hormone research was the Fearing Laboratory at Harvard Medical School's affiliated Boston Lying-In Hospital. A subsidy from Mrs. William Lowell Putnam, sister of the president of Harvard University, provided financial support for a fifteen-year investigation of the cause of eclampsia, a rare but often fatal complication of pregnancy. George Smith, an obstetrician-gynecologist, directed the laboratory in which his wife, Olive Watkins Smith, was the biochemist. The Smiths observed that progesterone levels dropped prior to the onset of toxemia, when abnormal fluid retention, increased weight, and heightened blood pressure severely endangered the lives of mother and fetus. Eclampsia is accompanied by convulsions and is usually preceded by the clinical signs of toxemia. The Smiths studied high-risk women with previous pregnancy losses and saw that estrogen and progesterone levels dropped earlier in this group than in pregnancies where there was no toxemia. From these observations, they postulated that DES could be given to stimulate the placenta to produce an increased quantity of natural hormones.

Smith and Smith launched a treatment regime based on their observation that specific dosages of DES at specific times in pregnancy altered the production of natural hormones and that the alteration improved pregnancy outcome.[14] In 1945 they enlisted 119 obstetricians in the United States and Europe to do clinical trials of DES in high-risk pregnancies. Between 1948 and 1954, seven papers reported data demonstrating that DES had reduced pregnancy accidents and produced babies who were bigger than the average for their gestational ages. DES seemed effective because both the women who received the treatment and their babies did better.[15]

None of these seven studies was "blind"; that is, the investigators knew they were giving DES to women who had some basis for pregnancy loss, such as diabetes. In research, a "control group" is composed of subjects similar to the members of the experimental group in all respects save those under investigation, so that the results of the experiment cannot be explained by extraneous factors. Three of the DES studies used no controls, and four used inadequate controls. None of the control women was treated at the same time as the DES group or by the same methods and personnel, although they were roughly the same as the treatment group in other respects—age, social class, risk factor, and location of clinic. DES received enthusiastic endorsement on the basis of these seven studies, although it is impossible to conclude from any of them that it was DES itself that made the difference.

It is known that special care and attention to high-risk mothers by people who believe strongly in what they are doing and in the likelihood of a positive pregnancy outcome may be enough to improve the outcome of the pregnancy dramatically. The high-risk category can include women who have many different types of pregnancy problems—threatened miscarriage, past or habitual miscarriage or abortion, previous stillbirths or premature births, toxemia, medical conditions such as diabetes and heart disease that increase the risk in any pregnancy, nutritional deficiency, or hormonal imbalance, to name only some. In a 1953 review of papers describing various treatments of thousands of habitual aborters, Arthur G. King showed that regardless of the treatment used, including DES, and regardless of the increased personal or medical attention given to these pregnant women, a successful outcome resulted in 60–62 percent of the cases. Smith and Smith had reported pregnancy salvage rates that were somewhat higher (72–74 percent) from the use of DES.

A nine-year study of 160 women with histories of "habitual

abortion" (three or more miscarriages) was conducted at Cornell Medical Center–New York Hospital by Edward Mann and first reported in 1956. These women were treated with psychotherapy alone from the time of pregnancy diagnosis; 81 percent delivered healthy full-term babies. Among the 19 percent who aborted again, anxiety and phobic symptoms preceded the miscarriage. Other doctors at Emory University reviewed records of 1,570 women with threatened abortion who were treated without hormones; 72 percent did well with only bed-rest and frequent checkups. E. D. Colvin and co-workers in 1949 reviewed the records of the 28 percent of the 1,570 women who aborted to see if DES or vitamin treatment might have improved the salvage rate. They concluded that most of these miscarriages could not and should not have been prevented because the blighted products of conception would have been badly damaged children. In their analysis, fewer than 4 percent of the pregnancies might have benefited from hormonal treatment.[16]

The only way to separate out the effect of DES from the more general favorable outcome of conservative measures is to do studies that concurrently compare two similar groups treated by the same personnel in the same manner except for the administration of DES to one treatment group—that is, to use controls. Ideally the treating personnel should be "blinded" so they do not know which women are receiving which regimen and hence are prevented from the unconscious tendency to treat the experimental subjects differently.

In addition to the seven studies reported above, there were seven controlled trials of the Smith and Smith regime between 1950 and 1955.[17] Four of these studies were blind and three were not. Four used alternate controls, one used simultaneous controls, and two used randomized controls.[18] The largest and best known of these trials was done by William Dieckmann's group at the University of Chicago, which compared the effects of DES and placebos given to 2,000 women during routine first pregnancies. This series reported that DES either did nothing or brought about a slightly higher prevalence of reproductive problems than were experienced by the women who did not take the drug. The conditions that were to be prevented by DES—prematurity and infant mortality—seemed, if anything, to be made worse by DES.[19] In fact, all seven of the studies that used sophisticated methodology showed DES to be at least ineffective if not harmful.

Smaller studies from the U.S. Navy Hospital (Crowder et al. 1950) and from Columbia's Presbyterian Hospital (Robinson and Shettles 1952) showed that DES did nothing to improve salvage rates in women with threatened miscarriages. A report to the Medical Research Council on diabetes and pregnancy summarized information gathered from nine hospitals in the United Kingdom which had followed the Smith and Smith regime with diabetic patients chosen on a randomized basis (Reid 1955). These high-risk women were no more likely to produce live, healthy babies than those treated with an inert tablet.

The Columbia investigators stated, "The public has been so frequently told of the virtues of this drug through articles appearing in lay journals that it now requires a courageous physician to refuse this medication. The mass of pharmaceutical literature extolling the wonders of this drug has also rendered most practitioners amenable to his [sic] patient's demands." They commented that miscarriage occurs for so many reasons that it is illogical to assume only one cause and to suggest that DES is the one and only treatment.

Yet, the conviction of the drug's efficacy was so great that no attempt at a blind control or randomized clinical trial for various types of high-risk pregnancy was made by the proponents of DES therapy. The research methodology was available by 1948, when the first anecdotal series was reported.

Prenatal patients who have lost babies and women desperate to conceive a child are groups from whom it is difficult to withhold a drug that the physician thinks might be helpful. This possibility can lead clinical investigators who are responsive to their patients to overlook the absence of proper trials.

Dieckmann designed his studies in conjunction with the Smiths. They agreed with his treatment regime but disagreed from the start with his extrapolation of the DES treatment to normal pregnancies. They had claimed that their therapy was "no panacea" and was specifically indicated only for women who had lost previous pregnancies. Dieckmann apparently studied DES in routine cases because he had noted in practice the increasingly widespread use of DES for normal women. When Dieckmann presented his work at a scientific meeting in 1952, the Smiths and some of their followers repudiated his results, claiming that they had no relevance for high-risk mothers and that DES was never meant to be a cure-all for everyone (Dieckmann et al. 1953, discussion pp. 1075 ff.).

Between 1950 and 1961, *The Physicians' Desk Reference,* a primary manual for practitioners which collates information supplied by drug manufacturers about their products, never mentioned the negative findings of the seven controlled studies; rather, it stated that DES was useful in preventing accidents of pregnancy.[20] By contrast, the *Merck Index,* published by Merck and Company, in 1960 stated that DES had *formerly* been used for prophylaxis of preeclampsia, premature labor, and other late complications of pregnancy. The 1958 *Modern Drug Encyclopedia and Therapeutic Index,* which was not related to drug companies, mentions no usefulness for DES in pregnancy.[21] By the late 1960s, six of the seven leading textbooks of obstetrics had concluded that DES had no effect in preventing spontaneous abortions in any group of patients. Nevertheless, it has been estimated that as many as 100,000 pregnant women per year received DES for at least fifteen years after it was shown to be ineffective.[22]

Thomas C. Chalmers, then president of the Mount Sinai Medical Center, New York City, analyzed all the DES studies and cited DES as an example of the power of the anecdotal report and of the resistance of medical practice to the results of well-designed clinical drug research. He claims that if randomized clinical trials (RCTs) had been required for DES from the start, the drug would never have been used in pregnancy. Chalmers champions RCTs as the only way to minimize drug disasters. In the instance of DES, such trials would have shown the ineffectiveness of the drug even before its long-term dangers were discovered (Chalmers 1974, 1975, 1983).

In 1970, gynecologists Arthur Herbst and Howard Ulfelder, and epidemiologist David Poskanzer, at the Massachusetts General Hospital, observed the almost unprecedented appearance of a very rare cancer of the vagina in eight young women, none of them older than twenty. Until that time, this rare clear cell adenocarcinoma of the vagina had been known primarily in women over fifty,[23] and the team of doctors was perplexed. It was the mother of one of the young women who suggested that perhaps her having taken DES during pregnancy was related to her daughter's cancer. Her hunch led to a review of the birth records of all eight patients, which showed that seven of them had a history of prenatal exposure to DES through their mothers (Ulfelder 1980). When the report of this correlation was published in April 1971 in the *New England Journal of Medicine,* the medical community was stirred, alarm ran through the media, and the FDA issued a drug alert to all physicians in the nation, warning them that DES was contraindicated for use in pregnancy (FDA 1971).

DES was originally recommended for pregnant women who had been unable to bear children because of severe medical illness or diabetes and for those who had had repeated miscarriages. If, in fact, DES had helped these women to bear healthy infants, even the small incidence of cancer observed in 1970 might have been considered by these women, their physicians, and the FDA as a risk worth taking. Its usage, however, was widely extended to women in whom risk was slight or who had no apparent problems at all. While the Smiths had cautioned that DES was "no panacea," it was treated by other physicians as just that, and given to "make normal pregnancies more normal." DES became a routine part of the quality care that private practitioners gave their predominantly middle-class patients, including their own wives. Considered the best possible pregnancy enhancer, it was even included in vitamin tablets for pregnant mothers. The original rationale—that DES was useful in preventing toxemia—had been lost in the shuffle. Once Herbst and his colleagues had published their findings, the drug was disapproved for use in any pregnancy.

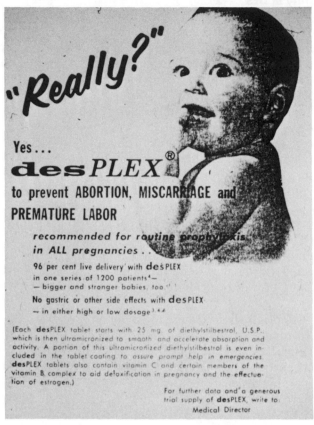

This ad appeared in a prestigious obstetric-gynecologic specialty journal in the 1950s. Note the happy, healthy baby and the recommended use of DES for all pregnancies. Note the references: (1) Canario, E. M., et al. (1953), *Am. J. Ob. Gyn.* 65: 1298; (2) Gilman, L., and Koplowitz, A. (1950), *N.Y. St. J. Med.* 50: 2823; (3) Karnaky, K. J. (1952), *South. Med. J.* 45: 1166; (4) Peña, E. F. (1954), *Med. Times* 82: 921 and *Am. J. Surg.* 87: 95; (5) Ross, J. W. (1951), *J. Nat. Med. Assn.* 43: 20 and (1953), 45: 223. Peña's series of patients is inflated by 1000; he actually reported on only 200 cases. Canario et al. used the Smiths' population and DES alone, not desPlex. We have not found any evidence for the statement that vitamins C and B "aid detoxification in pregnancy and the effectuation of estrogen." Neither Karnaky nor Ross used desPlex, so their patients could not have reported on "gastric or other side effects." Note also that the latest reference is dated 1954, yet no reference is made to the 1953 Dieckmann paper demonstrating that DES was ineffective for normal pregnancies.

Did DES do any good at all? We know for certain that DES, when given to normal women, at best did nothing and at worst increased reproductive wastage, as demonstrated in the clinical trials by Dieckmann and others. There was never an adequate large-scale randomized clinical trial of DES with problem pregnancies. Small, controlled studies concluded that DES was ineffective treatment for threatened abortion but failed to achieve public notice or to generate further research. The research methodology used in the original studies that established DES usage would not be acceptable now as the exclusive method for drug approval.

Our present understanding is that there is no consensus that DES did anything for toxemia. Some obstetricians still claim that it helped;[24] others are sure that it did not.[25] There are no data about which everyone agrees. If babies were going to be premature because of an underlying disease of the mother, DES made them plumper so that their chances of survival of their early birth were improved by the additional weight.[26] A tricky point here is that the Dieckmann studies suggest that in normal pregnancies DES increases the likelihood of prematurity itself. In many of the Chicago cases, then, DES may have contributed to the very condition its weight-enhancing properties improved. The Chicago results, however, cannot be completely extrapolated to a high-risk population where the prematurity itself is an indicator of the disease process.

Had a low incidence of clear cell adenocarcinoma of the vagina been the only problem with DES, and had DES been surely effective in preventing pregnancy loss, a problem with a relatively high incidence, it might have been worthwhile to consider continuing the use of the drug in pregnancy in carefully selected cases. But it is a fact that most miscarriages are caused by problems of the fetus, not by maternal deficits, and DES was a treatment directed at improving the maternal milieu (Colvin 1950, King 1953). As it turns out, clear cell adenocarcinoma is only the beginning of the story (see chapter 2, below).

DES is not given to any pregnant mother today. Hormones, however, including DES, are sometimes given to prevent pregnancy or to help a woman conceive if she is having difficulty. DES, although not officially approved for the purpose, has been used at high dosages as a "morning after" pill for postcoital contraception.[27] Current medical philosophy is to give minimal hormones or drugs during pregnancy. But hormonal drugs given to induce ovulation and promote conception are still present in the body at the time of conception.[28] And it is not known whether such drug residues can affect the developing embryo.

2
The Historical Context

The introduction of any new medical treatment involves a complicated interplay between research findings, the doctor's personal experience, and the patient's needs. On many occasions in medical history, techniques or medications have been accepted on the basis of anecdotal reports only to be rejected later, after other reports have revealed them to be ineffective or harmful. There is no way to tell what might have happened with DES had the link to cancer not been discovered. Only after a cancer scare were the negative research results heeded; only then was the prescription of DES to pregnant women stopped.

The DES story thus unfolds in the context of the long-standing tension in medical history between public pressure for a cure and the philosophy that argues for the restraint that avoids harm. Indeed, the history of Western medicine can be seen in terms of a dialectic between the "primum non nocere" doctrine and the Promethean desire to know and to cure without limits. Both forces have been responsible for advances and setbacks in the healing arts. In general, the more extreme the therapy in either direction, the more problems eventuate. DES was a bold treatment. It came to be used to prevent the possible problems of pregnancy and thus to alter the quality of life, not merely to control or ameliorate specific diseases or defects. Its application in its time was a dramatic example of daring, of tampering with nature and expecting to save and cure. Its popularity was untempered by information from studies suggesting that it would not succeed.

According to neonatologist William Silverman, DES was one of some twenty-five treatments introduced in the 1940s and 1950s to save newborn infants. All of these treatments, Silverman says, are examples of "medical inflation," the phenomenon whereby an interesting therapeutic observation comes to be regarded as a full-scale remedy. Only two of these treatments—exchange transfusion and respirator support for respiratory distress—have led to sounder practice; all the others have led to therapeutic dead ends, wasted effort, or definitive damage.

Silverman considers the story of retrolental fibroplasia (RLF) a "parable" of medical inflation. RLF, a type of blindness in newborns, was first described in 1942. It took twelve years to realize that it was caused by the life-saving supplemental oxygen administered to premature babies during the first days of life. The mysterious affliction occurred most frequently in babies born in the most advanced hospitals. DES also was given by the most up-to-date physicians, and given to private patients, rarely to clinic cases. Both DES and oxygen were felt to increase the survival chances of premature babies; both have since been linked to devastating results in those offspring.

The viability of premature, low-birthweight infants became visible as a significant and widespread problem only in 1939, when birth certificates began to list the length of pregnancy in weeks and the baby's weight at birth. Statistical records kept at local and national levels set a numerical baseline for tackling the problem of prematurity. All the innovations Silverman studied were developed in the United States with the zeal that had been unleashed during the war. For example, Silverman quotes from reports of a treatment with detergent mist recommended for premature babies: "After a year's experience, this is an almost infallible weapon for combating neonatal asphyxia. It enables one to attack this previously discouraging problem with vigor, enthusiasm and confidence."

This remark typifies the unbridled optimism and lack of restraint that greeted new treatment regimes in the 1940s and

1950s. It was indeed a common pattern, as we saw with DES, to shift rapidly and almost automatically from a reasonable theoretical speculation to everyday practice and usage. In the postwar era, the spectacular success of penicillin and other antibiotics led the medical profession and the general community to encourage other bold explorations and other "inflations." "Wonder drugs" and "miracle cures" were lauded by the press, and people clamored for them. The public atmosphere made it more difficult to test the drugs adequately and to ask the ordinary questions about their effectiveness.

When Silverman actually tested the detergent-mist treatment, he found it utterly useless. The manufacturer predicted that Silverman's report would not hurt sales, and indeed his published account of the negative results he discovered had virtually no impact on pediatric practice. Amazingly, cautionary articles in medical journals had little effect on the popular press, which continued to publish glowing reports, or on the eagerness of individual doctors of the time to act vigorously. Silverman's report was published in 1953, the same year as Dieckmann's studies of DES, and the detergent-mist episode directly parallels the DES experience.[1]

There is one well-known incident in the care of pregnant women and unborn babies in recent history that illustrates how stopping the use of a drug or not prescribing it can be a far more heroic act than giving it. The drug Thalidomide, in general use in West Germany from 1957 and considered safe and helpful there, came under consideration in 1960 by the FDA as a medication for treating the nausea of pregnancy. The drug manufacturer had begun a pro forma distribution of the pills to a group of "investigating" doctors who were supposed to be testing their efficacy. There was no serious expectation that formal studies would be done by these physicians; nor was there any anticipation of serious opposition. A brief letter, however, had appeared in the *British Medical Journal* of 31 December 1960 describing possible neurologic effects on users of Thalidomide (cited in Silverman 1980a, p. 83). It was read, by chance, by Dr. Frances Kelsey of the FDA. She inquired thoroughly about the drug's effects and learned that grossly deformed babies with seallike limbs had been born to some mothers treated with Thalidomide. The drug was withdrawn from the market in West Germany in 1961, but only after thousands of babies had been born in Europe with severe limb abnormalities (see Taussig 1963).

Because of Dr. Kelsey, Thalidomide never got beyond investigational status in the United States. However, later efforts to contact patients in the United States who had received the drug were frustrating; more than half of the 1,258 physician-"investigators" who had been given Thalidomide by the manufacturer had no record of the drugs they had received. This incident stimulated the 1962 Kefauver-Harris Amendment to the food and drug laws, which tightened the requirements for drug approval. It set out much more rigorous testing criteria, so rigorous that now some researchers complain that it is difficult to do their work, although public interest groups think the criteria are still not stringent enough. What makes the criteria more stringent is the requirement to prove efficacy.

Randomized clinical trials (RCTs) are now regarded as the best way to study the efficacy of a new drug treatment. This method compares the new drug either to a previous treatment or to no treatment in two groups of people who are so similar and so randomly assigned that they could have gone into either the treatment or the "control" group. The crux of the trial is that the control or comparison group must be observed simultaneously with the treatment group so that a judgment regarding the efficacy of the new drug is *relative* to the efficacy of another accepted procedure or to no treatment.

Randomized clinical trials were known as early as the eighteenth century, when James Lind compared treatments for scurvy. Claude Bernard anticipated the need for such trials when he described the process of research in three steps: (1) observation, (2) comparison, and (3) judgment. Too often, especially in clinical situations, an observation is made passively—something is noted to work in a particular situation. Then the comparison, or second stage, is bypassed, and a judgment is reached. Such judgments are based on limited data, perhaps even a single observer's single observation, and can lead to fallacious conclusions. Epidemiologist John McKinlay (1981) contends that most medical innovations are fully adopted prior to adequate testing. Promising clinical reports are usually accepted by clinicians and institutions and by the public, are endorsed by the government, and become standard practice before RCTs are performed.[2]

Although great discoveries have evolved from unique serendipitous connections, scientific progress—especially in those sciences involving human beings—is more often based on relative, comparative, and probable connections than on absolutes. It is therefore far preferable in clinical research to make an active observation—that is, to note that a particular treatment seems to have an effect—and then to state a hypothesis that will be tested to see if the observation is constant over time and place and thus can be regarded as more than a random chance event.

The comparison step is the most difficult and therefore the most difficult to get clinical researchers to do routinely. Implicit in doing a comparison is the admission that one is looking for a probable trend, not a guaranteed cure. A comparison done carefully, as an RCT is done, means delaying the gratification of an apparent dramatic conquest of a problem in favor of finding that something may—or may not—be a substantial improvement in the overall care of that problem. The comparison is humbling; it substitutes probability for inevitability. Doctors, like most other people, prefer absolutely certain knowledge to the medical school dictum "never say never, and never say always."

William Silverman (1980a, pp. 21–23) gives an account from personal experience with one treatment for retrolental fibroplasia. A patient who had suffered six previous miscarriages delivered a two-pound, six-ounce baby at twenty-nine weeks' gestation. At age two months, the infant developed numerous and tortuous blood vessels in the retina—early signs of retrolental fibroplasia. Use of adrenocorticotropic hormone (ACTH) had once been recorded as a way to reverse this process, and the treatment was introduced here to slow the growth of the blood vessels in the connective tissue in the baby's retina. ACTH, which stimulates the adrenal gland, appeared to have a direct dose-related effect on the inhibition of abnormal blood vessel growth. The infant's eyes returned to almost normal, and when she had gained weight, her grateful parents took her home.

ACTH seemed to be *the* cure for RLF. Only after "considerable discussion and soul-searching" were two randomized controlled trials begun. Fifteen babies were treated with ACTH for two years, and eighteen others were observed but not exposed to the drug. Silverman reported that "uncertainty concerning the effectiveness of ACTH was not hidden from the parents, but none were asked to assume the agonizing burden to allow chance to decide on treatment vs. nontreatment." When the results were tallied after two years, the importance of such comparative studies was borne out. One-third of the ACTH-treated group developed blindness compared to only one-fifth of the untreated group, and there were more deaths in the ACTH-treated group. In observations sustained over time it became evident that early RLF changes spontaneously regressed to normal in most cases. ACTH not only did not contribute to this regression, but the treatment itself further endangered the infants.

The methodologies of RCTs grew out of trials of antituberculosis drugs conducted by the British Medical Research Council in the mid-1940s. The supply of drugs was limited, and necessity required that they be carefully applied in situations in which they could be most effective and least harmful. It is ironic that the very same Medical Research Council that developed the RCT had earlier funded the research that developed DES. Had the new RCT methods been required for the older research, DES might never have been made so widely available.[3]

By applying laboratory criteria to the clinical situation, the RCT methodology has recently been refined. The procedure now requires that there be a hypothesis or a preconceived idea that the trial will verify or refute. Random selection, preferably done by random number tables, is mandatory; each person in a pool of patients must have an equal chance of being chosen for each treatment. Just as coins do not fall neatly in the sequence heads/tails/ heads/tails, so true random allocation is never merely alternative assignment. The treatment is assigned blindly, so that preselection criteria do not affect the choice and the person giving the treatment cannot introduce a bias about the treatment. Only in this way can a true comparison of treatments be made and the effects of the new drug per se measured and separated out from other factors such as the therapeutic zeal of an investigator who wants to emphasize the value of a new treatment. By law, people participating in such drug trials must give informed consent, saying that they agree to take drug A or B after they have been apprised of the known benefits and risks of both treatments.

RCTs may delay valuable treatment for people who could use it, but they often show that a treatment is ineffective or not worth the risk of its side effects. The requirements for RCTs may seem to the consumers of medical care to be depriving them of urgently needed treatment; however, thousands of treatments are developed each year, and none is absolutely good or absolutely bad. Most new treatments turn out to be ineffective or to have unacceptable side effects. RCTs attempt to determine the limits of applicability of new treatments.

Resistance to RCTs also comes from clinicians working in the most desperate human situations—those helping to bring forth life or to save it. New chemotherapeutic agents for cancer are an example of drugs required by law to have efficacy tests with RCTs. Yet doctors feel pangs of conscience for withholding something that may prolong a life they are working hard to salvage, and they are understandably reluctant to await test results. Similarly, DES was an innovative treatment that seemed to have the power to bring live births to couples whose previous pregnancies had failed, and refusing to prescribe the drug may have appeared to be an act of cruelty rather than caution.

Drugs represent only one area of therapeutic intervention in which abuse may arise from what we have called medical inflation. Certain surgical and radiological procedures also began as innovations and quickly became common practice, continued for years after they were shown to be ineffective or even harmful. Tonsillectomies, for example, were routinely performed for several generations of children afflicted with moderate to severe sore throats and respiratory infections. Their use was rationalized as a potential cure for rheumatic fever and for speech and learning problems. Even today tonsils are removed indiscriminately, although definitive studies have shown that they have an important place in the immune system and that children may be far better off with them than without them. What finally seems to have slowed the practice of routine tonsillectomy was the discovery that children with their tonsils intact were less susceptible to poliomyelitis than children who had had their tonsils removed. As with DES, what stopped this widespread procedure was a dramatic correlation with a frightening though rare illness, not the painstaking scientific demonstration of its ineffectiveness.[4]

From the early 1900s until the mid-1960s, good medical practice included the use of irradiation therapy to treat patients with such benign disorders as enlargement of the thymus, tonsils, and adenoids; infections of cervical glands, mastoids, and sinuses; hemangiomas; and acne. Because the thyroid gland was located in the same area as these infected targets of radiation, it frequently received direct or scatter radiation during these treatments. Evidence has been accumulating since 1950 that suggests a relationship between head and neck irradiation during childhood and an increased incidence of cancer of the thyroid gland. Over one million children were irradiated for these benign conditions. The incidence of thyroid carcinoma in three large groups that were studied is 5 to 9 percent. The time elapsing between the irradiation and the cancer may be as long as thirty years. This delayed impact is similar to that of DES, but casefinding has been better in the instance of irradiation (De Groot and Paloyan 1973, De Groot et al. 1977, Wilkins and Sandifer 1979).

Medical inflation is by no means an inevitable consequence of all new drugs and medical and surgical procedures. Since World War II medical technology has vastly improved the quality and duration of life—for example, through pacemakers, radiation therapy for cancer, chemotherapy, dialysis, open-heart surgery, and bone marrow and other organ transplants.

In the aftermath of DES and other inflationary incidents, some new approaches to improving the outcome of pregnancy are more conservative, less technological, and less medically oriented. Nonpharmacologic techniques for labor and delivery have become more popular. Lamaze and Leboyer methods of unmedicated, natural delivery have developed along with technological advances in fetal monitoring. Calls for the cessation of cigarette smoking and alcohol ingestion by pregnant women have received wide public attention.

Such public health measures frequently have more far-reaching and more beneficial impact than dramatically innovative medical treatments, but they are rarely considered as newsworthy. Although advances in nutrition, water purification, and sewage disposal have saved thousands of lives in the past century, they have received much less publicity than new fashions in medical therapy. There are no heroes in plumbing. And it is far more difficult to change public and professional habits than it is to introduce a new remedy.

Passive, conservative, "do less" techniques are in no way incompatible with active, dramatic, aggressive procedures. Both approaches to medicine can be effective, and both contribute to the richness of options that characterizes American medicine. Chemotherapy and hospices are needed; public health measures and noninvasive techniques do not preclude major technological advances.

Some treatments that were popular for centuries were ultimately halted not because they were ineffective or because deleterious side effects and delayed reactions were discovered but simply because they were replaced by newer techniques. Bleeding, cupping, and the use of leeches and various poultices were all indiscriminately applied in situations where they did little if any good and sometimes did harm. Taoist sages sold Chinese emperors magical "immortality" pills made of unicorn horn and dragon bone, and such pills sometimes killed their recipients. But some of these techniques are still in use. For example, cupping has a place in modern Chinese medicine along with Western drug therapy. Maggots clean some wounds better than surgical techniques or modern antibiotics.

While twentieth-century medicine has formally rejected earlier traditions, it is susceptible to the same enthusiasms and pressures that were evident in pre-modern times. A modern doctor may shudder at such therapies as bleeding, which was prescribed for centuries with no evidence of salutary effects, but the fact is that DES was given to millions of American women in the 1940s, 1950s, and 1960s, and there is no evidence that it did more good for the average pregnant woman than bleeding had done. Had DES not been linked to cancer, we might be prescribing it still.

We must remember that the people who brought about the advances in medicine, including those involved in the development and use of DES therapy, were on the whole careful scientific investigators and competent medical practitioners. But competence and carefulness do not protect patients from the sense of grandiosity in all technological fields that is so characteristic of these times of postatomic moon walks and satellites in space.

Pendular swings between activity and passivity, thrusting and temporizing, have characterized medicine throughout history. New developments in the twentieth century are shifting the balance point between these extremes. The individual fantasies of patients and physicians about sickness and health, the relationship between doctor and patient, and the willingness to bend or suspend rational judgment have remained constant over time, but the scale and structure of medicine and science have changed radically in this century. Science has become an industry; the research establishment within universities, business, and government is on a scale that is unprecedented. The social forces unleashed by the size of these organizations and the ramifications of the treatments they develop are often beyond the power of the individual physician to control.

DES was one treatment that seemed within the control of the individual doctor-patient pair; yet it simultaneously connected the doctor to the frontiers of endocrinological research. No one imagined quite how powerful the drug was or how extensively it would be used. Its long-range effects have yet to be fully assessed. DES was prescribed to make nature better, especially to assist in the scientific conquest of aging and mortality, to create control over reproduction and sexuality. Mortality and sexuality are two central areas of human concern. The fantasies and expectations around DES touched the core of both of them.

DES was a unique wonder drug in that it promised to prevent mishap, not merely to cure illness. Traditionally, medicine aims to restore the balance of nature by healing the sick and bringing the organism back to its naturally healthy state. DES may have been among the first modern medical substances that seemed likely to improve upon nature, to prevent natural defects and unwanted outcomes from occurring in the first place. The shift in the 1950s and 1960s from prescribing DES only in problem pregnancies to using it routinely, even in normal pregnancies, reflects this change in attitude, though at the time no one appreciated how massive a shift this was. Medicine's traditional goal—to assist the natural processes of life and healing—was replaced with the notion that the forces of nature themselves are subject to control. DES became a means by which life itself could be mastered. It could help create life, then maintain youth and inhibit aging. It promised to be an elixir of youth, the goal of an eternal human search.

"Hot flashes" and atrophic vaginitis in menopause and vaginal inflammation in the post-menopausal woman are causally related to a decrease in naturally occurring estrogens. The ovaries produce less estrogen as aging occurs. DES became a way to stop the inevitable aging process by supplying in pill form what nature could no longer provide in sufficient quantities. Thus a youthful vagina, skin and metabolism could be retained indefinitely. Despite a great deal of controversy and concern, the prescription of DES and other substances in what is called "estrogen replacement therapy" is considered customary practice today. Osteoporosis, a thinning of bone, is a condition of post-menopausal women, often treated by estrogen as well as by calcium, fluoride, vitamin D, and exercise (Quigley and Hammond 1979). The risks of estrogen use, which include endometrial cancer, are considered by many physicians and by their patients to be outweighed by the benefits of greater comfort and bone strength. The promise that DES will conquer the effects of aging and restore a woman's youthful sexual vigor bears with it an implicit denial of change and of death, ideas fraught with conflict and anxiety for every-one. Some enthusiasts have recommended that every woman past forty take DES to stem the tide of time and inhibit normal aging (R. A. Wilson et al. 1963). Centuries ago monkey glands and beeswax were prescribed for the same purpose!

Breast feeding declined in popularity in the 1940s, and DES was useful as a simple inhibitor of mothers' milk supplies. Before the development of DES and other lactation suppressants, the new mother who could not or would not breast feed suffered from engorged and inflamed breasts for days and could rely only on ice packs and cloth bindings for relief. Mothers who do not nurse resume their prepregnant breast size sooner and may re-gard this as enhancing their sex appeal. DES thus performed another social function: it supported the cultural ideal of sexual attractiveness by preventing post-nursing breast changes.

Much of the DES story has been portrayed by feminist writers as an example of male doctors doing something thoughtless and harmful to women. Gender-related issues are important to an understanding of reactions to DES, as we will discuss in subse-quent chapters. But the climate that produced DES existed for many other medical phenomena that were not all gender-related.

Throughout history, people have attributed illness to the un-seen and unknown and have attempted to solve the problem by eliminating these mysterious influences. Special power and mys-tery have been ascribed to organs of reproduction—particularly female organs, which are hidden from view and for a long time poorly understood. The ancient Greek concept of the "wander-ing uterus" (*hustera*) was developed to explain "hysterical" symp-toms; an inability to swallow, for example, was attributed to the uterus having wandered to the throat. Sweet-smelling remedies were developed to coax the uterus back to its usual location and foul-smelling ones to encourage it to abandon an abnormal posi-tion and thereby reestablish health.[5]

The ovaries were seen as the basis of neurosis for a time in the nineteenth century, and their removal was a recommended treat-ment for mental illness. And as we have noted, female hor-mones—estrogens—are substances that by definition elicit "oistrus," or powerful sexual feelings, even though this linkage does not apply for human females. Even in the early twentieth century, castration (removal of the testes) and removal of the ovaries were experimental treatments for psychosis. Charcot and his colleagues recommended and used ovarian compresses for the treatment of hysteria until the mid-ninteenth century. Clitoridectomy was practiced as late as the 1920s in the United States as a treatment for compulsive masturbation and for orgasmic dysfunction. And, astonishingly, in 1981 DES was prescribed to control masturbation in mentally retarded boys, although masturbation, like pregnancy, is not a disease but merely a natural process about which some people have conflicted feelings.[6]

Hysterectomy, surgical removal of the uterus, is also a popular medical solution to a varied and sometimes vague group of "female problems." Everywhere the procedure has been studied, the conclusion is that it is performed more than is necessary. The treatment is offered frequently with the statement, especially for women in post-childbearing years, that the uterus is a "useless organ." The continuing use of estrogen by post-menopausal women, despite the risk of uterine cancer, is similarly justified by the argument that the uterus is after all dispensable and can easily be removed.[7]

Consistent with the notion of disposable organs, partial vaginectomy, removal of the inner third of the vagina, was briefly recommended as the treatment for DES daughters at risk for vaginal adenocarcinoma (Sherman et al. 1974). Fortunately, "prophylactic" vaginectomies were performed only on a relatively few DES daughters who showed early adenosis. But some of the less mutilating procedures commonly used on DES daughters—cautery, laser treatment, excision, "weeding," conization—may reflect the same conviction: that removing the damaged part solves the problem. A decade's close surveillance has shown that most of these surgical interventions were unnecessary.[8]

DES was developed and became popular because of the universal human wish to control the mysteries of our own sexuality and mortality, and it was immediately caught up in the nexus of its historical moment. Dodds predicted that the confluence of commercial benefit and the promise of youth would make this sex hormone successful. He did not predict the physical damage and personal distress the drug would cause. No one anticipated the extent of its usage. No one can yet say for certain what it accomplished. And no one yet knows the full extent of the damage it caused.

3

An Event in the Human Body

The first article statistically linking DES with vaginal clear cell adenocarcinoma in daughters exposed *in utero* appeared in 1971 (see Herbst et al. 1971). Since that time articles and radio and television programs about DES have appeared steadily in the medical and popular media. There have been studies of mothers and offspring, both male and female, as well as papers that speculate about the effects of DES on body tissues and about the pathological conditions associated with its usage. Some articles trace the natural history of DES usage in particular populations. Others discuss new treatments and the prevention of problems that may arise following the use of DES. A government agency, the National Cancer Institute, maintains an information exchange that distributes updated medical reports to physicians and the general public.[1]

Much of the medical literature is confusing to the lay reader. There is a lot of technical jargon; some reports contradict others, both in content and in the degree of concern they express over risk. This chapter presents a guide through the maze of medical thought about DES exposure and attempts to present the controversies, dilemmas, and paradoxes as they exist more than a decade after the initial startling presentations.

The chemical substance DES is a potent nonsteroidal synthetic estrogen. As we have noted, DES is stronger than estrogen derived from natural substances. It does not have the particular steroid structure that characterizes all naturally occurring estrogens and many body hormones, such as adrenal cortisone (see figure).

The original researchers on DES were quite correct in regarding this preparation as a fascinating and potent drug. It has had powerful effects upon the developing reproductive tract in boys and girls. It is connected with clear cell adenocarcinoma. It is associated with abnormalities of the structure of the cervix, uterus, and vagina, and with the condition called adenosis in the daughters of DES mothers, as well as with abnormalities of the male genitalia. There appear to be fertility problems for both males and females exposed to the drug, probably resulting from these structural changes. DES may even have an effect upon the developing brain before birth. This raises many interesting questions as to the direct action of DES on tissues, its delayed action on the body, and its interaction with other substances present in the body or ingested in food or drugs.

Why did exposure to DES contribute to so many different kinds of effects? First, the unique chemical structure of the DES molecule interacted with the developing cells of the embryo anatomically and biochemically to cause certain changes in the reproductive tract of the fetus. Second, DES functioned as an additional estrogen, participating in the natural hormonal interrelations within the body.

The first mode of action, the unique chemical structure, is understood even less than the second, the estrogenic function. No one knows exactly how the DES molecule did what it did to induce the developing embryonic tissues to follow an unusual course. It may well be that complete answers to such questions must await research with more refined investigative techniques, such as electron microscopy, histochemistry, and the immunochemical methods now being used in cellular biology.

Any explanation of the action of DES would have to account for both the teratogenic and the carcinogenic effects. "Teratogenic" literally means "making monsters." In common medical parlance, however, the term simply refers to the cause of any congenital malformation. The teratogenic effects of DES resulted from its influence upon cellular and structural develop-

Steroid
    fundamental structure

Estradiol
    an estrogen

Testosterone
    an androgen

DES (diethylstilbestrol)
    synthetic estrogen

ments in the embryo so that anomalous cells and formations occurred in people exposed in utero. DES is broadly called an embryopathic agent—that is, one that may cause structural and functional changes in the embryo.[2]

Fetal tissues are probably less sensitive to natural estrogen than the mother's tissues are. The protection afforded by this diminished sensitivity is incomplete, however; estrogen exposure does affect fetal organs, particularly the vagina, uterus, and breast in females and the prostate in males. Fetal tissues are even more sensitive to DES than to natural estrogen because the fetus has to use other biochemical pathways to deactivate the synthetic substance than the natural ones used normally to deactivate natural estrogen. In other words, fetal tissues are less sensitive than might be imagined but more sensitive than was ever predicted. Furthermore, the fetus probably becomes sensitized to all estrogens by DES exposure, a sensitization that may become important later in life.[3]

There has already been a wave of clear cell adenocarcinoma stemming from the transplacental carcinogenic effects of DES. Because DES sensitizes the fetal tissues to estrogen, it is feared that there may be further carcinogenic effects in the future. It is now known that estrogen-sensitized tissues may be more vulnerable to the carcinogenic effects of estrogen itself.[4] But as yet DES-connected cancers other than vaginal and cervical clear cell adenocarcinoma exist only in the realm of speculation, and there is no cause for alarm. It would, however, be prudent for individuals exposed to DES to have regular and frequent examinations, and it will be necessary for epidemiologists to follow this population for a long time before an all-clear can be sounded.

The DES treatment regime prescribed by Smith and Smith for high-risk mothers began during weeks five and six of fetal life (see chapter 1, note 14), and the dosage increased until the thirty-sixth week of pregnancy. Thus most of the first trimester of pregnancy, when embryonic development is most active and differentiation of structures is rapid, was blanketed with DES. The dosage schedules used in other studies varied somewhat, but all included significant doses during the first trimester and increasing doses at least until mid-pregnancy.

DES was supposed to provide a stimulus to the placenta to produce more progesterone and to increase the blood supply available to the developing placenta and fetus. But the preeminent concern of the researchers was with the favorable outcome of the pregnancy rather than with the mechanism by which DES itself acts on the developing fetus. None of the investigators anticipated the long-term effects that would ensue from exposing the unborn baby to DES.[5]

As we have seen, the carcinogenic effects of estrogen in animals were known even before the synthesis of DES, and recent work with mice confirms these early findings. DES was given to the mice by a regime comparable to that followed for humans. In the exposed group, many and varied tumors formed, and the incidence of tumors was directly related to the dosage of DES. The control group of untreated mice had no tumors. The evidence in human beings has never been this dramatic. In fact, there is as yet no animal model for clear cell adenocarcinoma. This means that it has not yet been possible to recreate in the research laboratory the same results that occurred in humans. The mice in the studies described developed many tumors, even one vaginal adenocarcinoma, but not of the clear cell type. Mice that are exposed to high levels of progesterone develop adenocarcinoma as they get older, but, again, it is not the kind of tumor that afflicted DES daughters.[6]

The six conditions in human females that have been causally connected to DES exposure are: clear cell adenocarcinoma of the vagina; adenosis; anatomical anomalies of the cervix; subfertility; carcinoma *in situ* and squamous dysplasia of the cervix; and breast cancer. Any theory of DES action would have to account for all these findings. So far, none has done so completely.

Clear cell adenocarcinoma of the vagina is the first problem that was discovered and the one most rarely detected in follow-up surveys of exposed women. Any individual DES daughter has a low risk of developing clear cell adenocarcinoma: 1/1000 through age 24, maximum for those born in 1951–53, and with a peak age of 19 for those born in any year. To put this statistic in context, it is important to understand that the total death rate from all causes for females between the ages of 20 and 25 is only 0.4/1000, and only 10 percent of these deaths are caused by cancer; 50 percent are due to accidents, especially automobile accidents. As of March 1984, just over 500 cases of genital tract clear cell adenocarcinoma were listed with the nationwide DES registry.[7]

The low incidence of this cancer among the several million DES daughters and the fact that some recorded cases of cancer do not have documented histories of DES exposure have been interpreted variously by different groups. Epidemiologists and pathologists working with the DES data say there is no question about the positive and causal association of DES and clear cell adenocarcinoma of the vagina. Gynecologists and clinicians working with the patients at risk understandably tend to emphasize the uncertainty of the association, interpreting the low incidence as perhaps revealing a less causal relationship, and one that can be explained by other carcinogens as yet undiscovered. We feel that the statistical evidence favors the causal-connection position of the epidemiologists. The difference in perspective, however, does not mean that the perceptions of the clinicians are faulty. People working with numbers see associations in large population groups. Those working with individuals wisely assess the risk of clear cell adenocarcinoma to a given woman walking through the office door as very small. A clinician working with a patient who has at most a one-in-a-thousand chance of getting clear cell adenocarcinoma is not so impressed with its danger. An epidemiologist who sees death from adenocarcinoma in an age group in which this form of cancer was previously unknown is appalled that it occurs at all.

To illustrate the complexity of the causal connection between DES and clear cell adenocarcinoma, consider the case of a set of identical female twins exposed to DES in utero. One sister developed cancer; the other did not. The one who developed clear cell adenocarcinoma differed from her sister only in her greater lifetime exposure to radiation and her more frequent viral illnesses (Sandberg and Christian 1980). This might suggest that one or both of these factors in conjunction with intrauterine exposure to DES gave rise to the cancer. Yet intrauterine development can be different even for twins who are identical genetically; for instance, one may show a malformation at birth that the other does not have. The development of all diseases reflects an interplay of many exposure factors, host factors, and unknowns.

Adenosis is the name for the condition in which cells that normally line the cervix are found on the walls and surfaces of the vagina. The cervix is lined with tall cells that look like columns; hence they are called columnar—or glandular, since they also secrete fluid. The vagina and its walls are almost always lined with flat cells, called squamous cells, which are better able to sustain external stimulation than the fragile columnar cells. In adenosis, areas of columnar cells are found in the vagina and on the outside of the cervix.[8]

Before DES was given, adenosis was described as a rare patchy condition in 4 percent of human females and 4 percent of primates. These figures came from routine examinations of women and from autopsy specimens. Adenosis has now been demonstrated experimentally in DES-exposed primates, where the condition is more widespread and is comparable to that of human DES daughters (Johnson et al. 1981).

As many as 90 percent of DES daughters have adenosis. When a physician, during a routine examination of a young woman, sees reddened areas on the pale cervix and vaginal walls that do not stain as they should, he or she will probably investigate the likelihood of DES exposure. Other markers of DES exposure are cervical erosion, ectropion, or eversion. This displacement of glandular tissue onto the outer cervix immediately suggests a DES history to the astute examining physician.[9]

Almost all instances of vaginal clear cell adenocarcinoma have been accompanied by adenosis. In five or six instances, a vaginal clear cell adenocarcinoma has appeared in an area where only adenosis was previously noted (Anderson et al. 1979). But adenosis is far more prevalent than clear cell adenocarcinoma, and, although it was originally thought to be a precancerous condition, in the vast majority of cases it heals and does not proceed to cancer (Burke et al. 1981). "Precancerous" is a label that means something different to statisticians and to clinicians. Calling something "precancerous" says to an epidemiologist that the risk of cancer is higher than normal, but there is not necessarily a reason for active intervention. Many clinicians reserve the term to describe lesions that can be actively removed in order to avoid cancer. Whereas the presence of adenosis does raise the risk of clear cell adenocarcinoma slightly, adenosis is not a lesion that can or should be removed. In fact, as noted, it tends to be self-healing and time-limited.[10]

DES daughters can be almost certain of having adenosis and, to a lesser extent, some anatomical variations. It is primarily for adenosis that DES daughters should be followed with six- to twelve-month checkups, unless symptoms arise requiring more frequent examination. Beyond the fear of adenocarcinoma, the presence of adenosis is significant because it indicates increased vulnerability to infection and infertility-inducing lesions and may be linked to other, as yet unknown, estrogen-sensitive cancers in females.

In women with adenosis followed over time, healing generally takes place by the third decade of life. This appears to be the natural history of these columnar cells that are abnormally located in the vagina: gradually they turn into squamous cells until the adenosis is completely gone. The process of conversion is called squamous metaplasia. But even when healing is complete, there may be some reason to continue examinations, since clear cell adenocarcinoma is a tumor originally found in an older age group, and there may be a second peak in its incidence. Cancers of the vagina, ovary, cervix, and breast are all estrogen-sensitive tumors and therefore theoretically could arise with increased frequency in the DES-exposed woman.

The cellular studies that seem to explain squamous metaplasia best suggest that during embryonic development the normal time clock of change is disrupted by DES. A natural process of growth is slowed down or inhibited by DES, and the usual and expected transformation of columnar cells to squamous cells during the development of the reproductive tract does not take place. Only in later life, under the influence of new hormonal spurts after puberty, does the transformation occur that should have taken place in utero.

The actual derivation of human vaginal epithelium is still controversial even after a century of investigation. It is known that estrogens stimulate the growth of tissues derived from the müllerian tubercle, an embryologic area that arises in female embryos six weeks after conception, when the embryo is only about ten millimeters in total size. In the traditional view, a pair of ducts—the müllerian ducts—elongate and then fuse to become the uterus and the vagina. The müllerian tubercle is a place where three different kinds of epithelial cells are in contact—müllerian, wolffian, and urogenital sinus. These cells, singly and in various combinations, have been considered the possible origin of the vagina. But much of the embryological work has been done on the rodent vagina, which develops differently from the vagina of primates. The human vagina is similar to that of monkeys, though it develops in a different time frame. No definitive understanding of the embryology of the human vagina has yet been reached.[11]

The origin of the ovary seems clearer. It develops from the initially undifferentiated gonad. The autonomous sex in mammals is female, and unless a Y chromosome is present to establish maleness, the gonad will become an ovary.[12]

Two sets of paired ducts, müllerian and mesonephric, are present in all embryos until the eighth week, when the sex of the embryo is established and the provisional ducts of the opposite sex—mesonephric in females and müllerian in males—regress and largely disappear. This occurs in the presence of circulating testosterone, the androgen or male hormone (see figure). It is not surprising, then, that the presence of the estrogenic substance DES, taken by the mother and passed through the placenta to the fetal circulation, can have such a profound effect on the hormonal balance and on the developing genital structures.

Estrogens have effects on systems other than the reproductive system, but these are less apparent in the studies on humans than in research with animals. In utero estrogen probably acts upon the hypophyseal pituitary secretory mechanism in the fetal brain, which controls endocrine regulation for the entire body (MacLusky and Naftolin 1981; McEwen 1981). Estrogens act on the skeletal system to augment bone development, which is the basis for estrogenic treatment of osteoporosis, or thinning of bones, in older women. They also have an effect on metabolism and on salt and water retention.

Cervical anatomic anomalies are malformations of the cervix and vagina. They have been reported, in different estimates, in 18 to 25 percent of DES daughters. The percentage varies according to the time in pregnancy when DES treatment was started—the earlier in the pregnancy, the higher the percentage. These malformations seem to occur more often in teenage daughters and less often in older populations, suggesting that—as with adenosis—improvement takes place spontaneously with age. Such malformations look quite different from the normal cervix and have been classified as collars, "hoods," "cock's combs," and pseudopolyps of the cervix and transverse ridges of the vagina. Young women followed for DES exposure may be alarmed to hear their sexual organs described by such phrases and may fear malformations far more radical than the structural irregularities that actually occur. Photographs, videotapes, or sequential drawings can help them to understand and monitor their condition. These anomalies of cervical shape rarely create difficulties for DES daughters, except perhaps in choosing contraception. DES daughters may wish to bypass hormonal contraceptives in order to avoid additional exposure to hormones. However, a misshapen or flattened cervix may prohibit the use of a diaphragm, and a small uterine cavity may rule out an intrauterine device.

Subfertility is the most recently discovered problem in DES daughters and is currently the cause of both concern and controversy. When Bibbo first published a comparison follow-up of the patients in Dieckmann's Chicago studies, she suggested that DES-exposed daughters were less likely to become pregnant than unexposed controls. Since the mothers who were given DES and those who were given placebos had been alternately assigned, and since none of the women in the original studies was known to have reproductive problems, the fertility problems that showed up in the DES-exposed daughters could not be ascribed to simple inheritance. The nature of the subfertility may be related to DES-associated changes in the reproductive tract (Bibbo et al. 1977).

In 1977, uterine structural abnormalities were demonstrated in DES daughters. Kaufman used an x-ray procedure, called the hysterosalpingogram, to outline the inner shape of the uterus and tubes with a dye. The normal uterus looks like a pear with a Y-shaped inner cavity. DES daughters had a smaller than normal uterine space with constricting bands within the uterus, which was frequently shaped like a T. The DES group which had the T-shaped uteri usually had other changes also, such as adenosis in the vagina and cervical structural malformations. It is likely that the uterine anomalies developed from embryonic interference in the same way as the better-known and more visible cervical and vaginal changes. There may also be microscopic differences in the lining of the T-shaped uterus that are not apparent to x-ray techniques but may contribute to fertility problems and to the increased menstrual difficulties described by some exposed daughters.[13] Recent studies suggest that there may be alterations in the structure and function of the fallopian tube as well in DES daughters (DeCherney et al. 1983; Newbold et al. 1983a, 1983b).

Conception rates are approximately the same or slightly lower in DES daughters than in controls, but everyone agrees that there are major differences in the ability of DES daughters to carry a pregnancy to completion. Herbst, the first to note the association of DES with adenocarcinoma, concluded that there are large differences between DES and control women in their ability to achieve full-term live births. There are more nonviable outcomes and premature births for DES daughters (Herbst et al. 1980). Barnes and her co-workers, in a pooled fertility study from the DESAD project, found "no difference" in fertility or menstrual patterns between DES and unexposed women, but there were far more pregnancy losses in the DES group.[14] DES-associated reproductive failures include spontaneous abortions, tubal pregnancies, premature babies, stillbirths, and repeated pregnancy losses.

Why there is more pregnancy loss for DES daughters is not completely clear. Diminished cervical mucus at the time of ovulation may contribute to lower conception rates. The unusual shape of the lining of the uterus and the misshapen cervix probably contribute to tubal implantations, to premature cervical dilation, and to early labor. A rather grim series by Berger and Goldstein (1980) of referred DES-exposed individuals and their partners who were trying to conceive showed an uncorrected fertility rate of only 66.7 percent; this compares to an expected pregnancy rate of 90 percent in one year for average non–DES-exposed couples who use no birth control.

These statistical estimates do not speak to the experience of an individual woman or to the pain of a fertility problem. DES daughters are still in the peak reproductive years. There is little doubt that, statistically, they can expect more difficulties with reproduction than their non-exposed sisters. While not every DES daughter will have problems, many may have some difficulty conceiving and may need special care to remain pregnant and to deliver a healthy baby.[15]

The DES daughter must arrange for vigilant gynecological care. She should have regular and frequent examinations by a physician she knows and trusts. Unless there are symptoms prior to menarche, these visits should begin at the time of her first menstruation. Before the age of menarche, vaginal examination is psychologically and physically traumatic and may even require general anesthesia. Such loss of consciousness only increases the sense of helplessness and fright. Not only is there the feeling "something is wrong down there," but one is being handled by strangers and is unable to be aware and in control. The procedure may thus amplify alarming fantasies that are already rampant in the premenarchal girl. Of course, any DES daughter will be more anxious about her first examination than other young women. The first menstrual period goes along with emotional and physiological changes that can make the examination easier to perform. Yet this initial examination, even in optimal circumstances, will require sensitive preparation and sometimes mild sedation.

In routine screening examinations of a DES daughter, it is now generally recommended that a Pap smear, bimanual examination, and direct visualization of the cervix and vagina be done. The diagnosis of adenosis changes can be better followed if acetic acid or Lugol's iodine stain are used. Where there is suspicion of a problem, DES daughters should be referred to medical centers with the capability for more sophisticated monitoring of tissue changes. A major monitoring method, but one that is not available at all medical centers, is colposcopy, which allows a magnified view of affected areas in the vagina and cervix.[16]

As we have noted, DES exposure substantially correlates with clear cell adenocarcinoma of the vagina, adenosis, cervical anatomical changes, and subfertility. Clear cell adenocarcinoma is the most dangerous and least prevalent condition; adenosis is the most prevalent and is usually benign. Cervical anatomical changes probably correlate with uterine changes and may contribute to some of the reproductive problems seen in DES daughters.

Three areas that remain controversial are now being investigated: (1) the possibility of future female genital cancer, including cervical, breast, and uterine cancer; (2) the behavioral effects due to the impact of DES on the developing brain; and (3) the effects of DES exposure on male offspring.

Squamous dysplasia, carcinoma in situ, and *cancer of the cervix* are not yet epidemiologically connected with DES exposure. It is theoretically possible, however, that the process of squamous metaplasia, the changing of columnar cells into squamous cells, which causes the healing of adenosis, may not stop at that point but might move on to dysplasia, changes in cell structure, and neoplasia, or cancer. The large area of transformation and the transformation itself potentially increase the risk of squamous cell neoplasia in DES-exposed women. DES daughters are not yet in the mid-life age group where cancer of the cervix is typically seen, but there is speculation that they will be at higher risk as they age.[17]

Breast cancer among mothers who took DES during their pregnancies has been presented as a potential risk, and the actual extent of the problem is being measured. If DES is a general human carcinogen, we would expect to see an increase in all tumors in those who have taken the drug, especially in tumors sensitive to estrogen. DES could be a risk factor contributing to the current high prevalence of breast cancer. The epidemiology of breast cancer is being studied worldwide; the United States and Canada have over six times the rate of breast cancer as Japan, and four times as much as Europe. Within the United States, age-adjusted incidence rates appear to be stable. Breast cancer occurs with increasing incidence from age 25 to age 50; after 50, it continues to increase with age but at a slower rate.[18]

The Mayo Clinic Center studied 408 DES mothers as part of the DESAD project. Although the conclusion was that there was no increased incidence in this group, the sample is too small and the study too short-term to conclude that breast cancer will not become a problem for DES mothers.[19] The University of Chicago follow-up study found an increased—though statistically insignificant—number of breast cancers at younger ages among DES mothers compared to a control group.[20] The Chicago finding was the basis of the DES Task Force Alert about breast cancer in 1978. More recent reports from the University of Chicago suggest that the differences between the DES and control-group breast cancers have been narrowing with time, suggesting decreased cause for concern.[21] A British follow-up study of diabetic women suggests an increase in breast malignancy among those treated with synthetic estrogenic hormones. But the conclusions are questionable because the sample was very small and the study included as "tumors" lesions that may not have been malignant.[22]

There has been speculation as to whether DES works as a hormone to stimulate the breast tissue to cause cancer or whether it is a directly carcinogenic molecule. It is known that as DES binds to the DNA in the cell nucleus it acts as a direct carcinogen.[23] DES as a synthetic estrogenic substance also acts as a hormone in the body, especially on the breasts and the reproductive tract. Therefore, women who took estrogens like DES in the past should probably be especially cautious before adding even low-dose estrogens during menopause so as not to increase the risk to themselves (Weinstein 1980).

Uterine tumors, especially endometrial cancer (cancer of the lining of the uterus), show increased incidence with each decade of life and are known to be estrogen-sensitive. It is therefore possible that DES-exposed mothers and daughters could be at greater risk in their later years for this cancer.[24]

Brain and nervous system: During fetal development hormones have an effect on the nervous system. Animal studies have found that sex hormones seem to play a major part in differentiating male and female so-called sex dimorphic behavior. At least in rodents, DES can reach the brain in a biologically active form to exert its organizational effects (see Herbst and Bern 1981). It may do so in primates and humans as well. Sex-dimorphic behavior measurements have included energy expenditure, social aggression, parenting preparation, affiliative contacts, gender-role labeling, and grooming.

Ehrhardt and Meyer-Bahlburg are currently studying the long-term effects in humans of prenatal DES exposure on mental health and psychosexual development, including both stereotypic gender behavior and emotional difficulties. They have written a critical review of the effect of fetal hormones upon the central nervous system (1981, pp. 1312–1318). Gender identity seems to be based on postnatal influences, but sex-dimorphic behavior and temperamental sex differences seem to be modified by prenatal sex hormones. The role of the in utero endocrine milieu has not been conclusively demonstrated, and its study is methodologically complicated.[25]

An unexpected and worrisome finding from a British follow-up study is that psychiatric illness, especially depression and anxiety, was reported twice as often among DES-exposed subjects as among the nonexposed. The general practitioners who reported the psychiatric status of their patients did not know about the patients' DES history.[26] The finding cannot be understood by any factor other than in utero hormone exposure.

All these correlations of later behavior with hormonal effects upon the developing brain are as yet inconclusive, but their implications are of such significance that they require thorough investigation and adequate explanation.

Males: Follow-up studies of physical changes in males are difficult to do and to interpret. The methodology of such studies is complex because there is no single condition to follow, such as adenosis in females. Bibbo's first follow-up at the University of Chicago (Bibbo et al. 1975) found lower sperm counts, anomalous structures, and lessened fertility in DES-exposed males. Epididymal cysts were significantly more frequent, as were testicular underdevelopment and small penises. (See also Cosgrove, Benton, and Henderson 1977; Driscoll and Taylor 1980; Hoefnagel 1976.) Further follow-up, however, has not substantiated the 1975 reports, and there does not seem to be a significant difference between DES-exposed and nonexposed males in these conditions.[27] While other surveys have suggested more anomalies and lessened fertility in DES sons, these have not yet been conclusively demonstrated; further study is required of the effects of DES on male anatomy and of the genetic endowment from their fathers. At the time of this writing, there are reports in the literature of greater than expected testicular cancer in DES sons, and a registry has been established at the Tufts-New England Medical Center.[28]

In sum, it is clear that DES influences the development of the fetal genital tract, and it is possible that it affects the fetal brain as well. Not all the long-term effects are known, either for the mothers who took the drug or for their offspring. The uncertainties about these effects can leave both patients and doctors with a sense of deep unease and helplessness. Learning about DES exposure may be traumatic; living with it requires patience and vigilance.

4
A Quiet Trauma

From the beginning, a central problem with DES has been how to understand what happened. The DES event has engaged a wide range of specialists: biochemists, endocrinologists, pathologists, oncologists, epidemiologists, public health officials, sociologists, and legal scholars, as well as obstetric and gynecologic physicians. It is our contention that the DES phenomenon needs to be analyzed and understood as a whole rather than divided into a dozen different specialist perspectives; for this a central concept is necessary. We believe that it is within the framework of the concept of psychological trauma and the terms appropriate to it that the entire DES experience—especially the responses of the physicians who gave it, the women who took it, the offspring who absorbed it, and the medical community as a whole—can be understood.

Trauma is a complex phenomenon, both as an initial event and in its aftereffects. Interestingly enough, it may be the one psychological phenomenon that, when carefully studied by observers of many different psychological schools, has resulted in consistent observations and methods of treatment.

To understand how DES has been traumatic, we need first to illuminate trauma in general. The DES experience, while it can loom as catastrophic to those affected, may be so widely diffused in its impact that it may not necessarily appear traumatic to a casual observer. As psychiatrists, however, we are accustomed to recognizing the traumatic force of past events—even of events that may not have been experienced (at least consciously) as traumatic at the time—and tracing their relation to current symptoms and behavior.

The whole gamut of experiences associated with trauma has been seen in the aftermath of DES. The insults inflicted by DES are social and personal, external and internal, public and private, sudden and enduring. Emotional responses ranging from total denial to mature reintegration can be seen among all those concerned: researchers, physicians, mothers, children, and the community at large. In this chapter we will describe the nature of trauma, to create a backdrop against which we will then explore the peculiarly poignant trauma of the DES mothers and their children. In later chapters we will discuss the trauma of the obstetrician and of the medical community when the magic hormonal elixir turned out to be poison.

The word *trauma* comes from the Greek word for wound, or external assault. Psychologically, trauma means an event or experience that is unexpected and undesired; an event that disrupts, temporarily or permanently, the sense of bodily or psychological integrity. A trauma is the stroke of the hammer that cracks the previously intact crystal and so reveals the hidden structure. The loss of a leg in a car accident, for example, is always traumatic; many patients continue to experience the "phantom limb" syndrome, the painful presence of the absent limb. The pain from the severed limb represents both neurological and psychological attempts to maintain a feeling of wholeness of the body image as it had always been up to the time of the loss. It takes work and time to get used to this loss. If, however, the loss of the limb has been anticipated and carefully discussed with a physician, as sometimes happens in cases of chronic diabetes, it may result in a range of less psychologically traumatic responses. The extent to which the trauma is reduced or avoided will depend on how well the person has been prepared for the surgical removal, the meaning and value of the amputated limb, and the adaptability of his or her personality.

For everyone, sudden and acute loss is always psychologically disrupting to some extent. Adjustment to loss, whether of a part of one's body or of a part of one's mental world, follows a distinct pattern that has been carefully studied. The sudden loss of a child, a friend, a parent, of a life plan or a dream, can be disruptive in the same way that an external wound can be. The healing of all trauma, whether the unexpected loss of a limb or a loved one, an external physical disaster or a psychological assault or some combination of the two, requires the capacity to mourn the experience as a loss and to come to terms with a world that is no longer what it was before.

In addition to acute, one-time external assaults, there are also situations of chronic trauma, such as internment in a prisoner-of-war or concentration camp, where the experience of being assaulted and helpless seems endless. Here the cumulative effect of unanticipated horrors upon the mind makes grieving nearly impossible until the entire situation has ended. The extent to which survivors of such experiences are able to redefine their existence after the traumatic series of events depends on their adaptive capacities, the specific nature of the trauma, and the availability of support during and after the period of maltreatment. Concentration-camp victims who have survived extreme and continual trauma sometimes are unable to realize they are safe even years after their rescue. One woman who had been at Auschwitz, for example, continued to steal and hoard bread for her children; other survivors have reacted with terror to relatively minor events such as a fire alarm and a common illness. Delayed stress reactions and serious emotional disturbances have been observed clinically in a large number of Vietnam veterans. They feel guilty about their own survival, they have difficulty with attention, memory, and sleep, they go to great lengths to avoid activities that remind them of traumatic combat events, and when exposed inadvertently to events that symbolize or resemble the original trauma, they become deeply upset. This widely recognized pattern is called the "post-Vietnam stress syndrome."[1]

A consequence of all trauma is the emergence of a sense of deep personal vulnerability. Many things in daily life might be intensely frightening if we permitted our thoughts to dwell upon random dangers. We suspend these fears because it is so improbable that they will be realized, and the dangers are impossible to avoid anyway.

We have distinguished between acute and chronic trauma. Another important distinction is between solitary and mass trauma. In any loss or horror, of course, one is always ultimately alone, but it is quite different to be bereaved, for example, by oneself and as part of a family. Being injured alone in a freak accident is different from experiencing disaster as a member of an entire group that is assaulted. The Chowchilla bus kidnapping on 5 July 1976, the Buffalo Creek disaster on 26 February 1972, and the Coconut Grove fire on 28 November 1942 are instances of events producing mass trauma which has been carefully studied. Communal disaster is generally easier to bear than private crisis; there are opportunities for shared solutions in group experiences that do not exist in traumatic events that befall only one person. The individuals affected by group disaster also suffer privately, but they are less prone to the distorted thinking, self-blame, and guilt that characterize individual trauma (Terr 1979, 1981a, 1983a, 1983b).

Human beings take a certain level of security for granted. The ability to deny what might actually occur at any moment is part of what we call "mental health." Even physical health can be enhanced by denial in some circumstances: for example, heart attack patients who denied experiencing fear had fewer complications and were discharged from the hospital earlier than patients who acknowledged being frightened.[2] But in any acutely traumatic situation, the sense of order is disrupted and one's ordinary ability to deny possible catastrophe is lost. Acute trauma victims develop a feeling that the improbable can happen in any sphere since it has just happened. They may develop a sense, transient or more lasting, of being threatened and victimized, a feeling of being assaulted by a dangerous and hostile world, and even, ultimately, a suspicious and frightened stance toward everything in life.

This feeling of extreme vulnerability is so unpleasant and disruptive that the healthy person's mind often goes to extreme lengths to avoid considering the fragility of life and the transient nature of relationships. People tend to ignore and distort perceptions that could force them to such realizations. For example, in an attempt to hold onto the stability that a beloved relative provides, a child will avoid for as long as possible recognizing visual clues of the person's serious illness.

In sudden trauma such denial and distortion are not possible, so that the very foundations of a person's sense of reality are shattered, at least temporarily. The first response to such a traumatic loss or assault, therefore, is disbelief: "This is not happening. It is not true." Even those who struggle to accept the news frequently find it difficult to comprehend at first; there is an unreality to the event: "This couldn't be happening to me."

Disbelief represents the earliest phase of reaction to traumatic loss; it is the attempt to come to terms with something that is unbearably painful and in the face of which everyone feels so helpless. This form of denial seems to be universal; it is the beginning of normal grief and precedes later transformations.

As the reality of the traumatic experience gradually penetrates, the victim next begins to attribute blame, to concentrate with great intensity on who is at fault, who is responsible, in an attempt to focus attention outward. Fantasies of taking active revenge can be temporarily satisfying because they lessen the sense of passive helplessness.

Self-blame—often absurd and irrational—soon becomes part of the response. "It's all my fault. If I hadn't had that mean thought this wouldn't have happened. If I hadn't indulged myself and bought that expensive thing, this wouldn't have happened." The theme is: if I were better, good, more nearly perfect, less at fault, disaster would not have struck. The victim continues to seek a causative agent, first outside himself, then inside. Utterly unrelated "causes" may be identified, such as mean thoughts or selfish acts. While blaming himself would seem to increase the victim's pain, it is the normal response by which he decreases the more devastating sense of randomness and helplessness. Little children will say that if they had really been good, Mommy wouldn't have died. Whether or not there really is an external causative agent is entirely irrelevant to this process. It reflects the way all children think, and in trauma the child in all of us is reactivated.

As these phases of denial, blame, and self-blame pass—and in the healthy person they do pass eventually—the victim becomes overwhelmed with rage. These feelings too must be experienced and expressed. After the Job-like fury at the unfairness of the loss or injury, a period of deep sorrow sets in. This sadness, if and when it becomes tolerable, eventuates finally in resignation and acceptance of the traumatic event.

For some people there is a further stage in the grieving process. Beyond resignation and acceptance there is a transcending of the trauma, the emergence of a new organization of the meaning and purpose of life based on the reality that the trauma has occurred and has been accepted.

The pattern described here has been identified in individual responses to such assaults as rape as well as in massive natural disasters. The process of gradual acceptance does not progress cleanly and directly from one stage to another. The various phases reflect the way the human mind attempts to integrate into everyday life an experience that is altogether unthinkable and unacceptable to the person and his view of the world.[3]

Anyone can get frozen at some point in the grief process. Sometimes a significant depression will occur. Because of conflicts and problems from the past, fixation can occur at any one of the steps—denial, blame, rage, sorrow. This is because there is a congruence between the particular emotional constellation of one of these phases of the process and the person's unresolved psychological needs and conflicts. In some instances, a person does not progress because he required help that was not available at the time, or because his personal energies had to be used in other ways and there was simply no energy left for grieving.

Emotional maturity, external sources of emotional and material support, and the general character of the personality all affect an individual's ability to cope and adjust. A particular traumatic event can be more devastating to a small child than to an adult or even an older child because a child's sense of self and of reality is less established and his adaptive mechanisms are less practiced. If a child feels protected by a loving parent, however, the trauma itself will be minimized or even dismissed in the magical sense of safety that comes from the comfort of parental care. This was demonstrated by the greater mental health of children who were held in their parents' arms in the London Underground during the blitz of World War II than of children who were sent away from their parents to be "better protected" in the country. Without the parents (or parent surrogates), the young child is more vulnerable than an older person (Freud and Burlingham 1944).

It should be clear, then, that although the response pattern to trauma, whether acute or chronic, individual or collective, is universal, understanding an individual response requires a detailed grasp of that person's situation, opportunities, and capacities.

It is possible for observers as well as victims to distort the image of trauma for psychological reasons. The human capacity for empathy usually makes a noninvolved observer likely to identify with the feelings of the trauma victim. This identification may make the observer feel guilty because he has not suffered such a loss; or he may feel threatened by the sense that "there but for the grace of God go I." Observers may therefore wish to deny and avoid such empathic helplessness and pain. This may explain why the vast medical literature about physical trauma contains few discussions of the emotional impact of physical injuries.

Victims themselves may wish to avoid the grieving process and thus may reimmerse themselves immediately in their lives, seeking to rekindle the hope and optimism that sustained them before the trauma. If adaptation is only superficial and does not result from a thorough integration of the trauma, they will pay a long-term price for the pseudoresolution. One cannot judge the impact of an experience by the way people seem on the surface or even by their behavior. Paradoxically, those who appear to be the most severely affected and upset initially may be more fortunate in the long run because their distress may elicit attention and care and may give them an opportunity to discuss their feelings and become less isolated. Those who slip into a too rapid adjustment may fool themselves as well as others and may be more vulnerable to later problems than more overtly upset persons. Many concentration camp survivors appeared to be functioning very well as long as they were busy and active making new lives but became psychotic or developed severe somatic illnesses when they had to retire or when their children had grown and no longer required their care.

Finally, there is a wide diversity in adaptive responses to trauma, not only in regard to the phases of the grieving process, but in the style of the final adaptation. In large "warehousing" nursing homes, angry and rigid people tend to do better than gentle folk (Lieberman and Tobin 1983). In some concentration camps the inmates who proved most likely to survive were those who were skilled in conniving and manipulating or able to develop such skills under stress. Other survivors were gifted in helping to create cohesive groups that offered mutual support and thus lessened the potentially traumatic effect of their experiences. People with highly developed imaginations and the capacity for complex and poetic thought are less able to deny the precariousness of life and more prone to experience the deeper vulnerabilities that others can put aside. Such people may not do well under severe stress. A great deal depends upon how the stress interdigitates with the individual's imaginative life and support resources.[4]

The DES pill produced trauma in unique ways. DES as a medication is related to sexuality and fertility, to the past and the future. It touches on issues at the heart of the mother-child relationship. In all grieving, the childlike parts of us return, and we seek, literally and spiritually, the care of our mothers or of those who represent basic maternal care. But one of the most disturbing features of the DES experience is its isolating nature, because the usual sources of help are the very sources of pain. It is the providers of early tender care who have let down the DES daughters and sons—unwittingly, the mothers brought pain to their children; the physicians brought pain to their patients. The ultimate sources of help became the targets of all the feelings involved in mourning—denial, blame, self-accusation, rage, and sadness.

Despite its many complex effects, DES remains most powerfully connected with childbearing, which is both a profoundly private experience and a complex social event involving the extended family and the larger community. Childbirth taps a
woman's deepest sense of her own body, intensifies her relationships with her loved ones, and, in addition, awakens fantasied
communion with past figures who have been important to her. It
involves the continuity of the generations, in her mind and in
actuality. The trauma of the DES experience, then, follows from
the violations of feelings and relationships that are intensely private and based in the most essential expectations of trust. The
obstetrician, trained to deal with the simple, natural problems
that can occur in pregnancy, hardly expects or is expected to be
the source—however unwittingly—of disasters. The reproductive experience of the mother is obviously not intended to poison
the reproductive capacity of her children.

From working and talking with DES mothers and daughters,
we have come to see that the quality of the experience surrounding DES lies somewhere between a natural disaster and a bad
dream in which safe relationships appear uncannily menacing.
DES, an unnatural substance, touched the most natural process
in an area of being that is usually intimate and untouchable. In
pregnancy and birth, a woman's expectations of her doctor
should be for trust and nurturance; yet childbirth arouses her
earliest and most primitive fears. In the healthiest and happiest of
persons and families, this combination of external and internal
components of the DES trauma has brought up distressing and
brutal fantasies and long-buried constellations of conflicts and
concerns that had been solved quite satisfactorily in the course of
development.

The emotional trauma of DES exposure is great and is frequently extremely subtle. Observers who are not aware of this
trauma or do not seek to understand it are not likely to notice its
profound and far-ranging implications. Typical expectations of
researchers about the effects of trauma are based much more on
external disasters than on such personal and internal events.
There is a peculiarly threatening quality to a disaster that comes

from within oneself and cannot be seen. Indeed, the psychological consequences of DES can be far greater and longer-lasting than the physical effects. The majority of people affected by DES were not psychiatric patients but ordinary individuals who experienced a disaster. Most of them are urban, white, and middle class, accustomed to being in charge, not to being underdogs or injured parties. Unlike most trauma victims, however, they do not form a natural group.

The more a trauma concerns our children or aspects of ourselves we value, the more difficult it is to overcome. The lingering emotional impact of DES is related to the fact that the drug damages the most private places in the body and those central and preemininent emotional concerns of puberty and adolescent development for parents and children: namely, the sexual organs. A leg injury is less emotionally charged for most people than an injury to the brain or the eyes or the genitals. That leg injury, however, will be more traumatic for a ballet dancer or an athlete than for a desk worker. But every one of us has especially strong feelings about his or her sexual organs and reproductive capacities. There is also particular irony and horror for mother and child in the awareness that the bodily tissues DES was supposed to heal are the very ones adversely affected by it.

5

Mothers and Daughters

A son is a son till he gets him a wife.
A daughter's a daughter for all of her life.

Modern psychiatric knowledge might dispute this folk wisdom but would acknowledge that the mother-daughter relationship is intimate, powerful, and crucial to the daughter's emergence as a mature woman. It is fraught with possibilities for intense competition and greater hostility than obtains in cross-gender relations. Competition between father and son is more open, a socially accepted step in a boy's progression toward maturity. Women are socialized to subvert their aggressive feelings; thus the negative and hostile dimension of the relation between mother and daughter has fewer explicit outlets. This does not mean that relations between fathers and sons are easier, but it is easier for them to maintain distance between them, which permits a short-run solution to problems of rivalry and tension.

For both daughter and son, the mother is usually the first supportive and nurturing figure. This is not to say that the father cannot do the "mothering" if the mother is absent or otherwise unavailable or that his role as father is not crucial for daughters as well as for sons throughout their development, but the mother has traditionally been the primary object of attachment for both genders during the first years of life.[1] The son switches to his father for gender identification from his initial primary attachment to mother; the daughter switches to her father as love object but retains her gender identification with mother, who remains her model of what it is to be a woman. Her mother is her standard for relating to other people and for handling the whole range of human impulses and appetites. As the world expands, mother remains central for the daughter: she can have babies as mother does, and she wants Daddy as mother does. If all goes well in the relationship, if there is affection and tolerance between mother and daughter, the daughter will wait to become a mother—as her mother did—until she is grown up, and she will choose a man who shares her father's virtues.

The daughter will similarly model her experience of her body after her perception of her mother's experience. If mother is comfortable being a woman, comfortable with her sexuality and happy in her expression of it, her daughter will probably feel comfortable with her own developing sense of her sexuality. If mother is tense and conflicted about being a woman, seductive with her daughter as a means of easing her own sexual tensions and conflicts, the daughter will have problems with femininity.

By eighteen months of age, girls and boys already have a sense of their own genitals. From then on, at every developmental stage there is a new integration of the body image. Studies have shown that following actual physical injury or a traumatic loss of an important person, small children will experience severe anxiety that will be manifested as fears of bodily defectiveness and mutilation (Roiphe and Galenson 1982).

By adolescence, the genitals begin to be experienced as organs of relationship to other people as well as sources of private pleasure and future childbirth. The anticipated quality of those relationships for a daughter will have a great deal to do with what she senses are her mother's relationships and her mother's comfort and pleasure in sexuality. During the pubertal changes of menstruation, breast development, and altered body configuration, with the abrupt shifts in feelings and self-image they bring, the daughter's anxiety is reduced by her knowledge that mother went through it all and shares her experience. In ideal circumstances, the mother's presence through the course of these changes is a source of confidence and reassurance.[2]

DES undermines the bonds of experience between a mother and daughter and adversely affects the development of each. If the relationship between mother and daughter is good, efforts to cope with the inevitable confusion and uncertainty arising from the mother's DES history may be successful, even though painful. But the everyday strains of adolescence on both mother and daughter, with their alternation between rebellion and closeness, their loneliness and separations, are inevitably increased in a DES family. The sense that, unlike her mother, the daughter might not be fertile and able to have children and that mother, however unwittingly, was the principal cause of the daughter's problems intensifies the rivalries, anger, and competitiveness the adolescent girl normally feels. And it confuses her. The mother, who is her natural ally and is needed for support, is also the source of her pain.

The mother's response may include terrible guilt, denial, even paranoid rage; such reactions tend to isolate her further from the daughter who needs her. Anything that interferes with a girl's ability to identify with her mother, before or during adolescence, paradoxically inhibits her ultimate ability to separate from mother. Identification is usually a flexible tool: when it works well, it permits the daughter to rebel, to make her own way, to move away from too much intimacy with mother and strike out on her own. For some adolescent girls, the fact of DES exposure makes the bond with mother tighter, which inhibits this gradual individuation.[3]

The prepubescent girl organizes a sense of her own femininity and sexuality out of fantasies and sensations and stories and chatter with her friends—and occasional actual explorations. There have been no systematic studies of the impact of knowledge of DES exposure on emerging feminine identity in such a child. Other medical conditions that require early and frequent examinations of the genitalia are known to make the pubertal girl unusually self-conscious and confused about those areas, which are supposed to be sources of pleasure but yield discomfort and pain. The regular pelvic examination itself sets the adolescent DES girl apart from other girls who do not have such examinations until much later and have them less frequently. These examinations are repeated reminders that something may not be normal. The experience of younger children and adolescents can be expected to differ from that of adult women whose sexual identity had been formed before they learned about their DES exposure. For an adult woman, information about her exposure to DES is new and distressing material to be integrated into her already established sense of her womanhood; for a girl, the information becomes part of the very experience of becoming a woman.

It has been shown in studies of other traumatic events, such as the Chowchilla bus kidnapping, that traumatized children demonstrate less denial of their concerns and have persisting difficulty trusting adults and the world around them (Terr 1981b, 1983b). The ultimate impact of DES as a traumatic experience will depend on how the situation is handled by adults important to the developing child. The children will do best with honesty, matter-of-factness, and support from significant adults.

The saddest thing about the DES experience for young daughters is that it robs their adolescence of some of its magic. A girl's first visit to a gynecologist, which is often made in the company of her mother or a girlfriend, is a milestone, a sort of rite of passage that is long anticipated. For the DES daughter more than for other young women, this gynecological visit is laden with anxiety.

A DES daughter began visiting a gynecologist at age eleven, not for an examination but rather to get acquainted with the woman who would be her special doctor for a long time and to lay the groundwork for their future work together. The little girl was very brave and cheerful with her intelligent and sensitive gynecologist, the best response that could be hoped for in this situation. On the way home with her mother, however, as the distance from the medical center increased, her mature and adaptive attitude collapsed and she became a sobbing, frightened child curled up in her mother's arms.

Probably no one has a smooth passage through adolescence.

Adolescents mourn for their about-to-be-lost childhood, and most do so in turmoil. Adolescence is a time when the self becomes strengthened and defined through experimentation with the boundaries of experience, both in reality and in fantasy. It is the sense of limitlessness and omnipotence in the face of reality and separations from home that gives the adolescent years their sense of new horizons. DES disrupts the natural developmental process with a too-brutal reality too soon. It forces the daughters to consider issues of real death and real damage. The DES adolescent and her mother may have to mourn for the daughter's future loss in adulthood as well. There may be a premature closure on identity formation. Too many serious decisions must be made in response to DES at a time when youth and play should still contain a sense of infinite possibility.

> A twelve-year-old DES daughter nearing puberty anticipated her first examination with great dread. One day an elastic band on her ballet slipper broke, and with uncharacteristic fury and tears the girl yelled at her mother for "not letting me be a ballet dancer." As she sobbed, she told of the fantasy she had developed on the way to dance class. She would be such a beautiful ballerina in Class II that she would be rapidly accelerated to Class V and asked to solo in the *Nutcracker*. Being a prima ballerina had become an especially powerful compensatory daydream since she had learned about DES and had been anticipating a visit to the gynecologist. The broken elastic snapped her back to reality, where she was a good but novice ballet student. "I need to be a ballerina if I can't be a mommy."

Those DES mothers and daughters who openly express the fears, anger, and anxiety that are appropriate responses to trauma seem to adapt well. Those who persevere in expressing these feelings and fantasies recover more fully. They turn out to have healthier self-perceptions and body images correlating with their acknowledgment of the impact of DES. The women who remain more isolated tend to demonstrate more disturbed body images and are more likely to act self-destructively or to develop psychosomatic symptoms (Belsky 1978). Such women behave in a manner similar to that of other victims of trauma. In rape, for instance, repression and denial in the acute phases are associated with poorer outcomes than unrestrained expressions of shock and grief. Progress comes from talking with peers or attending self-help groups which encourage victims to ventilate their anger and share their feelings of violation, isolation, and helplessness. The fears that DES exposure engenders are best resolved by realizing that they are normal and warranted, and by sharing them.

Open communication of information and feelings seems to be most reassuring. Facts and photographs detailing the DES experience often help those involved to bear and master it. Many young women, for example, find that the opportunity to see their inner genitalia on videotape during a doctor's examination gives them a comforting sense of knowledge and control about what goes on inside their bodies (Burke et al. 1980).

For some daughters, appropriate and expectable fears related to DES expand into a preoccupying fear of cancer or a relentless focusing on bodily deficiencies and paralyzing fantasies about what is going on inside them. Such women will require additional expert help to put their concerns in perspective.

An attractive, poised, well-to-do college student came for treatment because of anxieties about her schoolwork. The academic concerns quickly turned out to mask depression, drug use, trouble having orgasms, poor self-esteem, and fears about social and personal intimacy. Her sophisticated physical presentation disguised massive confusion about her body's functions, disgust at the appearance of her genitals, and poor self-care—alcohol and cocaine use, poor nutrition, and excessive use of douches and perfumed genital sprays.

All these concerns were the subject of her psychotherapy. When she consciously acknowledged, perhaps in response to the treatment, that she was a DES daugher, all her self-hate and self-revulsion crystallized around her identity as a DES-flawed individual. Her fantasies and fears of genital damage, which were being discovered, explored, and understood in the thera-

py as deriving from guilt and shame over her ambivalent identification with her mother and her eroticized, guilt-ridden relationship to her father, now became anatomic reality to her, on
the basis of this one fact of personal history.

Painstaking work was done concerning the actualities of her
DES history, the condition of her genitals, the difference between the harm her mother had actually caused and the harm
she fantasized, whether she was adequate to attract a man of
her own, and whether she could separate from the parents she
considered responsible for her condition. Eventually all the
development she required was achieved in therapy—but always through the lens of DES.

Other DES daughters have experienced life-threatening illness
and responded with courageous resourcefulness.

A young woman of eighteen, a physician's daughter attending
a liberal arts college, developed vaginal cancer. She had radical
surgery to remove her ovaries, uterus, and vagina and subse-
quent plastic surgery to create an artificial vagina. She was able
to use warm, close friendships, her family, physicians, and her
own unconflicted intellect to support herself emotionally
through this crisis. She became interested in a career in medicine for herself during her own recuperation and rehabilita-
tion. At age twenty-five, she decided to go to medical school.

These two cases present an interesting contrast. In the first, the
mere revelation of DES exposure despite minimal physical pathology could have stalemated the emotional development of this
ordinarily neurotic woman had she not been in psychotherapy.
The second woman was not a therapy patient, nor did she need
psychotherapy for any underlying difficulties. She was able to
transcend the massive disappointments she suffered and use her
crisis in the service of her new career.

These cases are unusual because they represent so graphically
the two poles of relatively severe maladaptation and extraordinary courage, resilience, and sublimation. More often the response in a healthy woman is mixed. Joyce Bichler, in her book

DES Daughter (1981), reveals herself to have been a healthy, well-integrated person before her vaginal cancer was discovered. She eloquently documents how her personality continues to develop as it would have without the cancer but makes it clear that her emotional life is pervaded by traumatic losses and repetitive fears and memories that relate to her condition.[4]

Some women do not seem to make much at all of their DES history until special circumstances often cause it to erupt.

A 34-year-old married woman was in labor with her first, eagerly awaited baby. She and her husband were cooperatively relaxing and performing according to their natural-childbirth class instruction. The obstetrician examined her and found that the labor was not progressing well; he decided to give her some medication. Thereupon she became agitated, anxious, and increasingly irrational. She refused any medicine and began clinging to her husband and asking for his help against the "evil" doctor who was out to get her. The doctor had treated her infertility for five years and had known her to be a rational, pleasant, cooperative patient. He was naturally alarmed at this sudden change in behavior and called a psychiatrist to see the patient. In talking with the patient alone, the psychiatrist learned that she was a DES daughter, a known but not prominent piece of her medical history. Throughout the pregnancy she had been anxious not to repeat her mother's mistake by taking a drug that could influence her developing child and had not done so. When the doctor recommended medicine during labor, her fears of failing overwhelmed her. The doctor's apparently routine therapeutic decision was enough to awaken the mistrust and resentment she had felt toward her own mother and her mother's obstetrician. The psychiatrist's clarification of her feelings enabled her to accept both the medicine and the support of her husband and doctor. Labor and delivery of a healthy newborn proceeded without further events.

Very often the DES daughter will not experience anger at her mother for taking the drug. She will fully appreciate that her mother's intentions were absolutely the best, and a good relationship between them will help them through the period of uncertainty about DES changes and questions of future fertility. But a new stress situation is likely to lower the daughter's defenses and reveal her suppressed rage against mother's "evil" doctor and mother herself for putting her in this bind. It is a measure of this woman's stability that she required only brief clarification by the psychiatrist and the simple support of her husband and her obstetrician to reestablish her sense of reality.

In other daughters, anger toward the mother about DES will unite with an underlying and barely controlled rage against her that has characterized the daughter's feelings from earliest childhood. This anger will appear as extreme pathology.

A talented seventeen-year-old musician entered a music conservatory. Her history revealed her to be an anxious, dependent young woman who had a difficult time separating from a difficult and restricting mother. When she learned during her first pelvic exam at the college health service of her probable DES exposure, she became unable to practice, attend classes, or think of anything besides her defective body. She went home and saw her mother's obstetrician-gynecologist, who confirmed the diagnosis of adenosis. She dropped out of school and, with her mother's support, made the rounds of numerous gynecologists in her vicinity until she found one whom she convinced to do a prophylactic hysterectomy at age twenty-one.

Her concerns about her genitals had achieved delusional proportions, and she continued to have symptoms in her vagina. This led to frequent gynecological visits for biopsies, laser-beam treatments, and cautery.

At this point she was referred for psychiatric consultation. She proclaimed that her mother, by taking DES, had poisoned her body and that she would stop at nothing to remove all consequences of the poisoning. Immediate psychiatric hospitalization occurred.

Even without DES this woman probably would have become deeply upset, even psychotic, upon leaving home and would have been forced to return to the mother she hated and needed. Perhaps she would ultimately have required hospitalization in any case. Though her delusion formed around the seed of DES exposure, it could have achieved such magnitude only in a fragile personality.

A studious, religious, middle-class fourteen-year-old required medical hospitalization for her self-induced starvation. She had rapidly lost 30 pounds, became amenorrheic, and lost all her female body contours.

She was initially polite but cool to the consulting psychiatrist. Eventually she revealed that her obsessions about food centered around long-term struggles with her mother. These struggles had escalated in the past few years around her dating and emerging sexuality. She learned about her DES exposure when her mother, aware of her own exposure to DES, insisted that the girl have a gynecological exam. The daughter thought the mother was intruding upon her and looking for evidence of petting and masturbation.

When the gynecologist confirmed adenosis and explained its origins to this young girl, she became quietly enraged at her mother and determined that she would get revenge by starving herself. Prolonged psychiatric treatment was useful in allowing this girl to develop comfortable acceptance of her sexuality and achieve age-appropriate distance from her mother.

This case illustrates how learning of DES exposure can traumatically unleash massive bodily anxieties in psychologically vulnerable individuals who might otherwise have managed at least marginal adjustment had there been no physical correlate of their worst fantasies. The patient was one of seven anorectic teenage girls we have seen whose dietary obsessions began after they learned of DES exposure. We wonder whether the recent epidemic of anorexia in upper-middle-class young women could be demographically connected in some way to the maternal population which was DES-exposed.[5]

Women's capacity to create life gives rise to fantasies about their fecundity and power. Every culture has myths of the Magna

Mater and female seasonal symbols of fertility.[6] In the twentieth century, however, mothers have been singled out for their power to harm. They have, at various times, been deemed totally responsible for childhood schizophrenia and accused of causing all developmental problems of infancy, either through rejection or through overindulgence. The pendulum has swung back in recent years, but the milieu into which DES was introduced was one in which mothers were particularly aware of their power to do damage to their children. Child care manuals during the post–World War II baby boom were concerned with the psychological and physical vulnerability of children. Pediatrician Benjamin Spock reassured mothers that they knew more than they thought they did, but went on to imply that the attitude and behavior of the parents, but especially the mother, have a profound impact on the developing child.[7]

The sense of potential destructiveness is, of course, implicit in every relationship of caring: if I can help, then I can withdraw my help and thus hurt. What I can give I can take away. Certainly all mothers are conscious of the helplessness of their infants and their power over them. No normal mother wants to do harm, but all relationships have some mixture of positive and negative feelings, at least in fantasy. Mothers who took DES may even have done so because their physicians urged them to "do their best" for the unborn infant. For a mother who learns that out of love and a desire to give birth she may have caused harm, there is terrible pain.

A conscientious forty-year-old mother told of her experience on learning about the aftermath of DES. She looked at her healthy, radiant seven-year-old daughter and said to herself, "Oh my God, I've killed her!" All the work and pride she had invested in her daughter to that point, all her self-esteem as a mother, was momentarily shattered. She felt that this one wrong move, unpremeditated though it was, would destroy not only her daughter's health and happiness but her life. Her guilt was so great that she was determined to devote her life to gathering information about DES and informing others. This frantic activity distracted her from her daughter's current life and was probably worse for the child than the exposure to DES had been. Fortunately, this mother soon realized that she was overreacting out of her shock and fear and that there were more realistic and less dramatic ways to deal with the situation.

The reason this woman could eventually grieve for the harm to which she had exposed her daughter and recover had to do with the fact that she had always been quite comfortable as a parent, and the fear that she had damaged her child by taking DES did not resonate with any long-term anxieties about being a hurtful mother. But for women who are uneasy about their mothering, a not uncommon problem, DES exposure may become the focus of deep-seated ambivalent feelings.

A fifty-year-old, tense, constricted librarian also had a guilty reaction to DES. But she felt most guilty about her hostility to her teenage daughter. DES was seen as proof that she was a bad and destructive mother and that her daughter would do best not to heed her advice. Their poor relationship worsened after the DES exposure and its potential effects were revealed. DES also became a metaphor for the daughter's feelings of betrayal by her mother. Hostile silences characterized their relationship, and the daughter became sexually promiscuous in an effort to obtain from boyfriends the support, nurturance, and reinforcement of her physical, sexual self that she felt her mother had denied her.

Mother and daughter may have come to terms with DES exposure and collaborated effectively on medical care only to have the trauma poignantly reactivated around the daughter's reproductive life. Mothers typically feel affirmed when their daughters give birth. They experience their daughters' having children as reflecting a positive identification with them. DES mothers may fear that, because they took the drug, they have failed to equip their daughters both psychologically and physiologically to have babies. So for them the question of whether or not their daughters wish and are able to have children is particularly complicated.

A fifty-year-old woman entered therapy for depression related to menopause. It soon became clear that she was happily married and coping quite well with her bodily changes. She had, however, become quite preoccupied with her daughter and obsessed with her wish for a grandchild. As the story unfolded, the mother revealed that she had taken DES to have her daughter twenty-eight years earlier. She had become increasingly reattached to her daughter and saddened by the daughter's repeated miscarriages and inability to carry a baby to term. Her depression resolved as she understood her sense of guilt for her daughter's condition. She could then permit her daughter and son-in-law to resume their own lives and could commiserate more appropriately with their struggles and losses.[8]

Fears about sexuality are tied in with the particular emotional charge the DES experience has for everyone involved, whether she is the innocent victim or the unwitting vehicle or perpetrator of what she feels to be destructive forces. The fact that the genitals are the target of the DES hormone has provoked some unusual responses that, in our estimation, point to deeper aspects of the DES trauma, concerning DES sons as well as daughters.

The initial reports of DES-associated damage focused on female offspring (Herbst et al. 1971). It was five years before any follow-up study of DES-related effects upon exposed males was reported (Bibbo et al. 1975), and clinical follow-up of DES sons is still less thorough and more controversial than that of daughters.[9] We wondered why workers in this field did not consider male genital damage sooner, and whether the seeming absence of concern had to do with the difficulty both researchers and victims had in acknowledging potential genital damage in males. A DES son is quoted in *DES Action Voice* (June 1980):

"Why is it so hard to get DES sons to come forward? The fact is that men do not easily talk about genital problems. . . . In our society the stigma attached to genital problems totally threatens the male identity. If a man is impotent or sterile, he is made to feel less of a man."

Our culture is more familiar with castration fear in males than in females. We believe that the DES experience has shed some light on female concerns. The concept of "castration anxiety" is technically based on Freudian oedipal theory, which focuses on fears in the boy aged four to sex about penile castration by the father as punishment for the boy's sexual wishes toward the mother (Freud 1923, 1924, 1925, 1931). Castration anxiety is often generalized to refer to all anxiety about the loss of body intactness in males and females of any age. Since in the male body genitals are exposed, the castration fears of males tend to focus concretely on the loss of the penis.

Both men and women, however, tend to underestimate the impact of genital damage on women, as if—as Freud thought— they see women as already castrated. This leads to an inflation of the impact genital damage would have on males and a corresponding minimizing of the potential impact of such damage on women (Horney 1933). The frequency with which unnecessary hysterectomies have been performed on premenopausal women speaks to this point (see chapter 2, note 7). It seems to us that, in spite of our increasingly sophisticated understanding of female sexual development, our culture retains the view that intact male genitals are more to be prized and can be devastated more easily than female genitals, and the penis is valued for its symbolic significance even more than for its anatomic function. Both men and women participate in developing and maintaining this value system. As a result, both men and women tend to exhibit greater anxiety in the face of potential danger to the penis, because it is both more valued and more visible; thus there is also a greater tendency toward denial.

Women's relative ability to face and adjust to genital harm may reflect the fact that women are more accustomed to attending to bodily changes. Each month they anticipate and experience menses, and with it the expectation of menopause. All through life women have, in addition, at least some subliminal awareness of childbirth, with its temporary changes in contour and physiology. Males, by contrast, lack such experiences and are socialized from earliest childhood to idealize bodily integrity.

Recent psychoanalytic work throws a different light on the developmental value of the genitals. In people with anomalous sexual organs, the most valued organ is the one they are supposed to have, not necessarily the penis. Females born without a vagina yearn for a vagina and value that above all.[10]

Female castration anxiety, then, is not generally recognized. We refer here not to women's anxiety about having somehow been castrated or to the anxiety that males and females share about the general loss of body intactness, but to specific apprehensions about losing the female genitalia. When asked by an interviewer about fears that they had never expressed spontaneously, several young women exposed to DES said that their primary fear was of losing their vaginas (Belsky 1978). The interviewer found that the fear of organ loss was even more prominent than the potential loss of fertility. Everyone is most afraid of losing what he or she already has.

It may be that male physicians' tendency to grossly underestimate the trauma that even the idea of losing a female organ has for women is a means of mastering their own castration anxieties. Fears of losing their vaginas have powerful unconscious roots and strong emotional effects upon DES daughters. Some of them do not communicate these fears to their physicians, perhaps because of a sense of how frightening it would be to acknowledge their worst fantasies to someone with the medical competence to carry them out. It is also possible that the extent of their rage at the thought of such mutilation is so great that the thought becomes repressed.

There are, then, barriers to communication from the patient's side. Young women can be so fearful that they do not talk as explicitly and directly as they might, and their fear may be manifested as anger or indifference. It is important for physicians not to feel rebuffed by such anger or indifference but to understand that these are defensive responses. It is not the doctor's job to deal directly with deep underlying fears. However, knowing that these castration fears are universal, the physican can provide reassurance by commenting on the integrity and intactness of the patient's genital organs. Beyond anticipating her need for reassurance, the doctor should be able to elicit the patient's conscious concerns and respond to them.

Some physicians seem able to do this because of their personal characteristics. Others need special direction on how to take and share responsibility, be matter-of-fact, collaborate on future planning, and permit different kinds of women to express their feelings in ways that will enhance their sense of dignity and control. In this context, whether the doctor is male or female may make less difference than whether he or she is adequately empathic. On the other hand, for some patients, the mere fact that the physican is a woman, regardless of her personality, may elicit the trust and sharing of feelings necessary to deal with the impact of the DES trauma.

6
Patients and Doctors

It is impossible to understand the DES experience without a deep appreciation of the complex nature of the patient-doctor relationship. The special bond between patient and doctor is based in part on the earliest needs for body care and protection, needs that stem from infancy and childhood. This bond exists between all doctors and their patients, in health and in sickness. The patient, much as he or she may disguise it, on some level feels vulnerable and helpless when ill and wants to view the caretaker as omniscient and invincible, like the good mother of childhood who can take care of everything.

From this perspective, it is possible, though clearly oversimplified, to divide people into two groups: those who realize their potential helplessness in illness, and those who defend themselves so vigorously against this realization that they try to pretend they cannot be hurt. Interestingly, many physicians fall into the latter group. Some people even choose to become doctors as a means of denying their own vulnerability. They wish to stand firmly on the side of the healthy, with a comfortable gulf separating them from the sick and vulnerable. Physicians of this type will accept the power with which they are endowed by those who are dependent upon them because it reinforces their sense of strength. Similarly, there are many people who deny their vulnerability and have a very difficult time tolerating an infantile position, even temporarily. Such people make difficult patients. Others are socialized into the sick role; being an invalid both legitimizes and gratifies their intense feelings of dependency. There is a growing literature that deals with being a patient *qua* patient. Here, however, we have chosen to look at the patient with her doctor because that is the context in which DES was given.[1]

The dichotomized relationship of doctor and patient, in which the patient is sick and helpless and the doctor is the active helper, resonates with a universal childhood experience. There is a deep understanding between parent and child in which the child trusts that if there is something wrong with him, the parent will make him better. Implied in this understanding on the part of the child is a willingness to comply with the seemingly omnipotent parents. This understanding represents an early childhood pattern that reemerges throughout life at times of illness and stress. The patient expresses a wish, usually indirectly, to regress—to return to the stance of the young child. He or she wants the physician, like the mother in infancy, to take over bodily care and control. There are very few other public roles in which passivity is so culturally acceptable and encouraged as it is for the patient, whose capitulation and submission are expected. The caretaker-physician assumes the maternal role. He or she not only is concerned with physical care but also absorbs some of the patient's emotional anxiety over being ill, thus accomplishing the omnipotent feat of "taking care of everything."

Of course, most adult patients are unlikely to regress so completely, nor would it be beneficial for them to do so. At the fantasy level, however, and on both sides of the relationship, there is a pull to these extreme positions. Doctors often want and expect themselves to be able to take care of everything, and patients often wish to be cared for totally and are willing to follow any advice in exchange for dedicated maternal attention. More adult and egalitarian forms of collaboration between patient and doctor that permit the patient more self-reliance and encourage mutual respect, through study and even argument, are frequently abandoned under the stress of severe illness.

In this book, we talk primarily about female patients. We do not discuss the doctor-son or doctor-father relationship. DES fathers have not been studied, and little is known about their responses to the DES experience. DES sons are similarly slighted in this discussion. They have participated less actively than daughters in follow-up studies and have been less vocal about all aspects of DES. Generalities about physican-patient interaction, however, can apply to sons as well as to daughters.

For adult women, the obstetrician-gynecologist occupies a special role, beyond that of the physician who is used during crises and illnesses. Little girls, as we have noted, hear their older sisters and mothers talk about the gynecologist who performs health-maintaining functions for them when they are not ill. The women are preparing for sex, contraception, childbirth; they have questions about menstruation or concerns about breast and pelvic examinations. The gynecologist is an integral part of the young girl's evolving notion of what it means to be a woman, and he or she is connected to those dimensions of womanhood that are part of normal growth and development. The transfer of significant information often takes place in the context of the gynecologic visit.

It is no wonder, then, that the bonds between women and their gynecologists are strong and hard to break. It is more difficult for a woman to change her gynecologist than any other medical specialist, except perhaps her psychiatrist. The experience with the gynecologist evokes the earliest sense of self and body as established and organized around caretaking people in a social network. This is essentially and necessarily a powerfully conserving and protecting relationship. Therefore it also contains within it the potential to disrupt the basic sense of self and body.

The DES experience led to just such a major disruption in the gynecologist-patient relationship by violating the deep, unspoken bond of trust between them. In an effort to repair the bond or deny its rupture, patients tend to project the blame away from themselves and their physicians and to affix it to impersonal agencies, such as the drug companies or the FDA. This maneuver serves to preserve their self-esteem and their important ties with family and gynecologist. For all the physicians' fears of lawsuits, we have been unable to find a single documented case of a suit brought by a woman against her gynecologist for prescribing

DES. There are several hundred cases pending against drug companies.[2]

More often than not, fantasies, conscious and unconscious, form the unexpressed background that colors and enriches the person-to-person relationship between doctor and patient. The gynecologist-patient relationship is highly textured and extraordinarily complicated. The basic trust of the early mother-child relationship, which carries over into all doctor-patient relationships, transfers particularly to the gynecological one. For many women, the allusions to early maternal relationships are totally unconscious, lived out in their behavior toward the physician but never experienced at the level of awareness. Other women seem to have more access to wishes and fantasies about their physicians.

Women are on the whole more able than men to talk and joke about intimate matters such as gynecological experiences and other personal services. Joking about the gynecologist, typically done with affection and humor, serves the important purpose of acknowledging the significance and necessity of the patient-gynecologist relationship and, at the same time, its inherent embarrassment and strangeness.[3]

The gynecologist becomes a composite figure to a woman, and her positive and negative responses to him or her come from previous and present relationships with mother, father, husband, teachers, siblings, lovers, and even other doctors. "Transference" is the term psychiatrists use to describe the unconscious process by which internal experience based on past relationships colors and patterns current relationships. Whereas attitudes, fantasies, and such emotions as love, hate, and anger arise in present circumstances, their sources can be traced back to previous experiences. Transference can and probably does occur to some extent in every significant human relationship, and the historical transferential elements contribute to the richness of human interactions. Relations to parents and siblings are the earliest sources from which transference derives; those to teachers and doctors follow. If a boy has a warm and loving experience with his first-grade teacher which reinforces his good feelings about his mother, he will expect to have positive experiences with other teachers as he moves through school. A girl who has had traumatic relationships with her mother or teachers may well expect humiliation and injury ahead.

Gynecologists are caretakers; they also implicitly or explicitly grant or deny permission for emotionally charged behaviors. These functions will be more apparent and more tolerable in their interactions with some women than with others. Women who have experienced violation in particular tend routinely to expect and anticipate some violation in every human relationship they have. Others, similarly harmed, will simply not tolerate any violations at all. Some prefer a passive role and comply unquestioningly with any doctor who has an authoritarian personality; others seek an alliance with a more egalitarian gynecologist. This choice is frequently related to how respectfully the patient has been treated in the past and the extent to which her feeling of security is related to being ordered about rather than collaborated with.

Women inevitably have fantasies, conscious or unconscious, about their gynecologists, whether male or female. The intimate nature of this doctor-patient relationship inevitably gives these fantasies a sexual cast. Some women find a sexual fantasy preferable to the feeling of childlike dependency that is also evoked by this relationship. For most women, the sexual fantasies are elicited by male gynecologists and the dependency feelings by female gynecologists. But not always.

A married graduate student came for routine gynecological care to a supportive, matter-of-fact woman gynecologist. The patient, a shy young woman, spoke of her childhood in an isolated rural area and some of the stresses of school and her difficult family. She never referred to her developing relationship to the physician and seemed comfortable with her.

The student wanted an IUD (intrauterine device) for contraception, and when the appointment date arrived she came with her husband. She was very anxious and wanted him present during the procedure. When the doctor inserted the speculum, the woman became panicky and began to clutch her husband, saying, "What's she doing? What is she putting into me?" The doctor stopped, realizing that this terrified young woman was becoming paranoid. The patient continued to be accusatory and irrational. "What are you putting into me? What do you put into people?" The husband was apologetic and embarrassed. He said he had been surprised when his wife requested his presence. The doctor explained that the IUD would not be put in that day and that they could come back again to talk about whether she wanted to use that form of contraception. The gynecologist then sought psychiatric consultation on the case.

When the patient did not call back, the physician telephoned and set up an appointment for the husband, wife, and herself to discuss plans. The woman was entirely recovered, distant, and curt. Upon reviewing her notes, the doctor noted that the woman had revealed on routine history that she had a psychotic mother who had been quite seductive with her.

This reserved young woman was experiencing a homosexual panic in the presence of a female physician. At some level she must have anticipated difficulty, for she brought her husband, who had never before accompanied her to a doctor's office. It is unlikely that a male physician would have elicited these regressive terrors. Her fears were probably related to her psychotic mother and to fantasies and memories around the mother's seductive behavior toward her when she was young.

Although the relationship between a woman and her gynecologist is influenced by the lifelong unconscious experiences of each, it is determined primarily by the two personalities and their perceptions of present-day reality.

Many young women prefer female gynecologists. They feel closer to them as well as more respected by them. They expect more collaboration, more teaching and nurturance from women doctors, and this expectation seems to be commonly realized for women with younger female physicians. Sometimes older women gynecologists, trained at a time when it was rare for a woman to go through an obstetrics/gynecology residency, appear to be no less identified with masculine norms than their male colleagues are.

Along with the positive aspects of former and present relationships which contribute to the elaborately textured portrait of who the gynecologist is and what he or she represents for any particular woman, there are negative aspects as well. Real or fantasied experiences of assault, violence, rape, painful sexual encounters, intrusions, exposure, and prohibitions may also be transferred to the gynecologist. Serious trouble results for the patient whenever these unconscious experiences are given some reality in the gynecological relationship. When there is actual sexualization or sadism in the examination, the worst fantasied fears become underscored realities and conscious traumas. Explicit sex between doctors and patients does unfortunately occur, and such episodes shake the patients' sense of reality. Even encounters which involve no physical exploitation of the patient may have major psychological consequences if the doctor insensitively abuses the special intimacy of the therapeutic relationship, especially when the patient is impressionable, young, inexperienced, or regressed because of the examination situation.

> A sophisticated, curious, intelligent, and attractive sixteen-year-old had an interview with her mother's gynecologist to ask him some questions. He told her not to have sexual relations and not to get birth control. When she asked whether she should douche as her mother did, the doctor responded with a question: "Does your mom use one of those bulbs with a big nozzle?" The girl, who had seen the device at home, answered "yes," to which the doctor replied, "Mom just douches for jollies; she doesn't need it and neither do you."

This doctor had a contemptuous attitude toward the mother's sexuality and rejected the burgeoning sexuality of his young patient. The interview, potentially an opportunity for the transmission of facts by an authority, was reduced to a situation that reinforced sexual prohibitions. The girl found that her concerns did not get a hearing, and she was additionally troubled by the intrusion of disturbing thoughts about her mother. Teenagers are a particularly vulnerable group because their sexuality is so ambivalently viewed by adults. Often it is denied, as in this example, and sometimes it is overemphasized.

The DES experience devastated the doctor-patient relationship by subverting the structure of positive fantasy that underlay it. Understandably, many patients responded to the shocking news defensively and regressively. The competent, collaborative patient suddenly required repeated reassurances or, alternatively, in an unconscious effort to defend herself against such dependency, adopted a belligerent, defensive, and rigid posture. The physician, who had previously behaved maturely and responsibly, withdrew and isolated himself, thus altering an alliance that had developed over many years.

Let us take a closer look at transference feelings toward physicians and examine some of their sources. Most children "play doctor" in childhood. These games are often a child's first social experiences involving sexual explorations. They are also a condensed reenactment of a power relationship that children experience, for children visit the doctor at times of illness. For the child, the physician is *the* powerful person who "can make it better if anyone can." The physician's activities are a distillation and concentrate of parental caretaking responsibilities. Doctor games in childhood usually involve exploration of the genital area, so these elements of power and helplessness contain elements of sexual feeling as well (Simmel 1926).

The "lithotomy" position routinely used in gynecological examinations enhances these derivatives of power and helplessness from the childhood doctor games with their sexual overtones. The word "lithotomy" derives from the Greek words for cutting stones and was originally used in medicine to refer to the position assumed by the patient undergoing surgery to remove stones from the bladder. In the lithotomy position, typically used today for pelvic examinations in the United States, the woman lies on her back with her legs spread and her feet up in stirrups, thus exposing the external genitalia to full view. By contrast, Victorian women, for the sake of modesty, were examined standing up and fully clothed; they were examined blindly, under their skirts. The lithotomy position evolved to enable the physician to get a direct view of the vulva, clitoris, urethra, and anus and, with the aid of light and speculum, also to see inside the vagina and the cervix. For the patient on her back with her legs bent, the position is similar to the so-called missionary position in sexual intercourse. This parallel makes it difficult for most women to feel neutral and causes some to experience anxiety. Women may have feelings of humiliation when their spread legs are placed in stirrups; the limitation of motion also arouses feelings of helplessness and vulnerability. In addition to the actual vulnerability of the position, therefore, it may cause many suppressed feelings about the gynecologist to surface.[4]

The transference to the physician collects a remarkable number of early life experiences that ordinarily stay out of our consciousness or are repressed. The trauma of discovering the damage that DES might cause lifted this repression in many women. Transference feelings, usually part of the unconscious texture during life's activities, became exposed, and complex repressed dimensions of the doctor-patient relationship were uncovered. Unfortunately, this added a burden to the DES-exposed person and family. Paradoxically, the trauma was compounded by this emergence to consciousness of feelings toward the physician that were never intended to come into awareness. In the best of all possible worlds, unconscious transference feelings are examined only where there are particular problems to be scrutinized, and one examines them, by choice, with a therapist or counselor who has been chosen for such shared scrutiny.

DES-exposed persons are in a state of crisis at the time of learning about their exposure. They have to deal with the problematic and frightening practicalities of arranging for proper health care. They need to cope, but coping is made more difficult by the efflorescence of previously unconscious fantasies. The unconscious is timeless; different levels of development and fantasies from various times coalesce together. A woman experiencing a reawakening of these unconscious fantasies may feel and act simultaneously like an infant, a petulant two-year-old, a fact-finding ten-year-old, a rebellious teenager, and a mature, reasoning young adult. The DES daughter, mother, son, father, and physician each respond with feelings that come from different levels of development.

Many of the complexities of DES exposure are captured in the story—told in her own words—of a twenty-six-year-old DES daughter, an attractive, married professional woman.

I started seeing one gynecologist eight years ago—before I knew that I had this situation. And I felt pretty good about him. I saw him on a yearly basis. I was having a lot of trouble at that time, infections and pains, and just feeling like something was wrong—that my doctor didn't understand, that I didn't understand. But I would go to him and he would cauterize me, and it would make things better for a while. He told me that I had "erosion of the cervix" and that it was something a lot of women had. The word "erosion" sounded pretty weird to me, because that has a lot of connotations, like things falling apart. But I said, "Well, you know, the cauterization does make it feel better."

I moved away and went to another doctor and he examined me; it was a very quick examination. He said, "Gee, I think you are a DES child." I didn't even know what it was at that time. I had never heard of it. I asked him what it was, and he explained to me that DES was something mothers took not to miscarry, and I knew immediately that I was a DES daughter because my mother had a problem when she was pregnant; she was diabetic and had a problem miscarrying. So, I immediately went home and asked my mother and she looked at me and said, "Oh, you found out about it." And I went, "You mean you knew about this?" She said, "Yes, I heard about it a while ago but I couldn't face it." So I had some anger but I also understood that it was really, really difficult for her to deal with.

So I immediately went back to my gynecologist at home, who was her gynecologist as well, and said, "How come you haven't noticed this? You have been examining me for three years." He just said, "Well, it is something that is new, you know, let me examine you now." He examined me and he said, "Yes, you do have this situation but it is nothing to worry about. The incidence is very low." And I started asking him, because I have always been the type of person that likes information, likes to be spoken to in a way that I'll understand, what is going on with my body. He said, "If you would have cancer of the vagina which I am sure you won't—it's deadly. Come back in six months and we'll do check-ups every six months." I felt good about that. I felt, "Well, I'll be watching it, and he has a colposcope and that is what you need to check out this situation." So I just kept going back to him every six months. And every six months he'd cauterize me, as what he called "preventive." He examined me and told me, "Oh, everything looks the same, everything is fine. No problems."

Then I got a letter from a project that was being done at a large university hospital, being paid for by the federal government to observe DES girls. And I got all excited because I thought, well, I'd be in the mainstream of the research, I'd really know what was going on. (Also, before I continue, I think it is important to say that all the time he kept saying "don't worry" and he'd explain to me about cancer, there was a lot of fear involved, and it was like I just knew that I had something that nobody knew anything about, that there was no thirty-year study on. I was the thirty-year study, and sometimes that was really hard to deal with. Sometimes I have gone through cycles of being really depressed about it. I think the cycles are through. But it is just very hard always having an unknown.)

Anyway, I went to this project and was all excited about going there. And I enter a little room where you wait. Sitting on a table were two pictures of cervices, one with erosion and one without. This is a normal cervix, and this is an eroded one. And I am sitting there thinking, "This is what they have for me who is coming, who has this problem?" And I am thinking, "What about girls and women who are coming for the first time and really don't know anything about this? And here they are already being told something is normal and something is abnormal about them. And nothing is being explained."

Also, the doctor was a female doctor, which I was really excited about. Because I said, "Wow, a female doctor should really understand how we feel." I had seen my regular gynecologist the week before for my regular checkup. I went in and I just sat there on the table and she didn't say anything to me, and I just got ready to have the examination. And she starts to examine me. And she says to me, "Who cauterized you? Why did you let anybody cauterize you?" Like yelling at me for having that treatment done. And I was like, "Well, I've been seeing this doctor and that is what he does." And she continues to examine me and says, "Do you know you have an enormous cyst? It is gigantic!" And I am sitting there thinking to myself, "Oh my God, I have an enormous gigantic cyst. My doctor that I trust supposedly examined me a week ago. He didn't even notice this enormous cyst." I started to feel crazy. I really felt like the rug had been pulled out from under me. Like I had been working with somebody that I thought I had trusted, taking the best care of myself that I thought I possibly could, and here she is yelling at me and telling me that she found something he didn't notice the week before and it was enormous. Then she proceeds to tell me that she can't biopsy it now because of the cauterization. And so she says the word "biopsy" and that says to me, "Oh my God, she wants to do a biopsy!" That means she is looking to see if it is malignant. She thinks I have an enormous malignancy, a cyst! And I said to her, "Well, is this something you think is serious?" "Well, we don't know until we biopsy it." So I say, "When can you biopsy it?" "Oh, not for at least a month." So it is like I have to sit there for the next month wondering about this enormous cyst she found. Using words like biopsy to patients that have DES who are concerned about having vaginal cancer is really something pretty emotionally earth-shattering. It was for me anyway. And needless to say, it was like I was just totally devastated.

And I called up my old gynecologist and said, "Hey, I saw this doctor and she said I have this enormous gigantic cyst and

you just saw me last week." And he said, "Oh, come right in."
He examined me and said, "Oh yes, I see what she is talking
about. It is not enormous and gigantic. It is only this big." I go,
"Well, how come you missed it?" He said, "It is nothing to
worry about. It is not important."

So at that point, I felt like, "Wow. I have been seeing this
person for a while and he didn't mention this. She said it was
enormous and gigantic. Who should I believe? Like, how do I
know what is going on inside of me if I cannot trust the physicians I am seeing?" So I decided that I had to get another
opinion. So I asked some people about somebody else that I
could see and they recommended another doctor.

I went to see this other doctor and he confirmed that it was
indeed not enormous or gigantic and it was nothing to worry
about. Something that was really positive from this whole experience was that the doctor that I finally found sees me on a
yearly basis, takes videotapes and pictures so that he can compare yearly to see if there has been any change. Also while he's
examining me I watch the video so I can see exactly what he is
doing and he explains everything to me and he shows me this
and he shows me that. And that's been the most wonderful
thing because when people started talking about DES to me
and talking about lips on the cervix, I mean I really started
imagining all kinds of horrible things going on inside of me. It
was like all kinds of abnormalities and what is going on inside of
me. I think that just increases the fear and anxiety unbeliev-
ably. So to be able to see what it looks like and to have him point
out, he showed me my "normal" sized cyst, and he showed me
where he took the biopsies and how he took a Pap smear. I just
had the examination today and I said, "How come that is a red
spot there?" and he explained it to me. And I think that it has
just made me feel just so much more confident in following
this. Like I finally have somebody who talks to me like I am
intelligent and doesn't just pat my hand and say, "It's okay;
don't worry about it." You know, to be told not to worry about it
is one thing, but of course the anxiety is there.

I had little blame for my mother, like I kind of feel that I wouldn't be here unless she took the drug. Because she did have a history of miscarriage. I also feel like a real positive thing has come out of it in that I went off the birth control pill because I didn't want to be putting more hormone things into my body. My diet has changed completely. I eat a vegetarian diet now because there is DES in all the red meat that everybody eats. And I really feel that it is important that doctors start educating people about these things. So it really, you know, I think helped me in terms of my attitude.

This woman's narrative shows us many things. She attempted immediately to exonerate her mother, to understand her out of empathic affection, and she says, "I wouldn't be here unless she took the drug." She needed to justify her mother's use of the drug in order to ease her helplessness and diminish her anger. Were she to believe that DES had been unnecessary, her anger at her mother might be stronger, and the anger might extend to her mother's doctor for originally prescribing the drug.

One sees here the mother's guilt too, her wish to deny and hide. "You found out about it. I heard about it a while ago. I couldn't face it." The young woman could not readily turn to or get angry at this mother, who was already in pain. She did turn to her physician, partly as a mother surrogate. She was dependent on him and wished to be dealt with maturely and collaboratively. She felt confused and anxious in the face of his indirect explanations and ominous references to cancer. Despite all his obfuscation, she knew that she "was the thirty-year study" and confessed that "sometimes that was really hard to deal with. I have gone through cycles of being really depressed about it. It was just very hard having an unknown."

She was very excited to have a female doctor; very likely she hoped for the sharing of information and feelings she could not get from her guilty, denying mother or her patronizing male physician. She expected a great deal from a woman physician: "Wow, a female doctor should really understand how we feel." So her disappointment at the doctor's alarmist and insensitive responses was intensified by failed hopes of collaboration and ma-

ternal nurturance. What then follows is an all too familiar account
of the hazards of being a patient. Confused, blamed, disarmed,
she finally found a physician who attempted to communicate with
her in clear ways with pictures, facts, and a timetable and allays
her anxieties in the context of an empathic relationship. "That's
been the most wonderful thing . . . to be able to see what it looks
like . . . somebody who talks to me like I am intelligent." It was
important to her to feel that her mind as well as her body was
being treated respectfully.

Beyond the relief of being able to share her feelings with a
trusted physician we see her attempt to transcend the DES experience. Her changes in diet, drugs, and attitude have a poignant
touch of rationalization but nonetheless reflect an attempt to
learn from and overcome the source of her trauma.

Her recitation virtually catalogues the fears common to DES
offspring. When people began talking about DES to her, her
vivid imagination went wild—"lips on the cervix," unknown and
horrible things going on inside her. Vague and insufficient explanations only increased her fear and anxiety. Even the word "biopsy" was "pretty emotionally earth-shattering . . . I was just totally
devastated."

At a time when such regression and unleashing of repression
are to be expected, it becomes especially important that physicians collaborate with their patients rather than patronize them.
The setting of the gynecological examination and the trauma of
the DES disclosure may enhance regression, but it remains possible to counteract the backward pull by mature interaction between patient and doctor. With the stress of the DES discovery,
many transference responses to the physician emerge. Recognizing and understanding them can permit the doctor to bear the
burden of these transference responses lightly, not to take them
personally, and thus to be more effective with his patients, as was
the last physician in this example.

A thirty-year-old teacher had known of her DES exposure for
ten years and had been remarkably able to work with her mother and her mother's obstetrician to monitor her adenosis pre-

ventatively. She chose to use birth control pills, had been sexually active and adjusted, and was pleased with her work and her marriage.

She and her husband closely planned the time that she would discontinue contraception and they would start a family. Much to their dismay, she did not become pregnant the first year. The couple was evaluated for infertility and a probable T-shaped uterus was found but nothing specific to account for the delayed conception. The physician prescribed clomiphene, a powerful fertility drug. This made her anxious, reminded her of her mother's experience, and raised questions in her mind about the drug's long-term consequences that no one could adequately answer. She reluctantly took the clomiphene and became pregnant. However, the pregnancy was an ectopic (tubal) pregnancy which required emergency surgery and loss of her fallopian tube.

It was around this life-threatening event that her defenses broke down and her relationship with her long-time doctor became fraught with resentment, mistrust, and accusations. She had, until this point, felt that she was an active collaborator in her own health care, a feeling her doctor had supported. But when she was rushed to surgery, anesthetized, and lost part of her body as well as her pregnancy, feelings of helplessness and despair emerged. The physician sensitively encouraged her to be active in her expression of sadness by sharing his own grief about her loss and his sense of uncertainty about any future pregnancy. Together with her husband, they discussed the risks and benefits of various treatment approaches and made specific plans to attempt another pregnancy while considering adoption.

In this case, the relationship between the patient and her doctor minimized regression and supported her coping capacities. The primitive fears about bodily integrity and the aggressive feelings that began to emerge in the crisis subsided with his acknowledgment of her pain and loss, which strengthened her sense of adult mastery.

Sexual and aggressive transference feelings are especially complicated. Children are aware that their mothers and fathers are sexual beings in ways that the children themselves are not. They recognize that parents have experiences as yet unavailable to them. Each child experiences transient sexual longings for both parents. For the sake of the individual's development and for cultural survival, these yearnings must be set aside or repressed. This is a universal truth for both children and parents. Many an adult woman continues to experience guilt for her infantile sexual wishes, particularly when her relationship with her parents has been less than satisfactory. This guilt may prohibit her from expressing anger in general, and about sexual subjects in particular. Unfortunately, the prohibition frequently extends to situations in which it is entirely appropriate to feel anger, such as DES exposure.

Difficulties in expressing anger and rage are quite common among women in our culture and are reinforced by powerful social forces. Women often believe that to be loved and lovable it is best to be cooperative and compliant. As a result, any angry feelings they have are accompanied by guilt and anxiety. They therefore suppress these feelings in order to view themselves, and be viewed by others, as "good girls," good daughters, and, later, good mothers. Without doubt, women collude in this stereotyping. It is their reluctance to show anger, even to question or disagree with authority, that many DES mothers emphasize in retrospect. They recall being oddly unquestioning of the doctor's suggestions.

An intelligent, active woman, herself a health professional who had done research on prenatal development, questioned the advisability of her taking any pills early in pregnancy. Her obstetrician became more forceful and said, "I am advising you to take DES; are you questioning my advice?" The woman became frightened and guilty about her anger toward the doctor, backed down, and became a compliant patient. Later she regretted having taken the DES.

She was less angry at the doctor than at herself for having colluded with him.[5]

Sometimes the inclination to comply with the physician is inter-
rupted by a trusted intimate.

A thirty-eight-year-old teacher reported that she had taken
DES only briefly early in her pregnancy with her seventeen-
year-old daughter, a wonderful girl with whom she had no
particular problems. She herself had been an unsophisticated
young woman, too shy to ask questions when her obstetrician
recommended she take DES during this first pregnancy. On a
visit to her own mother in rural Maine, she told her mother
about the pregnancy and the doctor's advice, whereupon the
future grandmother became irate and said, "I know from my
own experience that pregnancy is a natural event and you
shouldn't bother with any pills." She flushed the DES down the
toilet with such determination and a sense of "mother knows
best" that her daughter felt there was no point in arguing with
her.

In situations of inadequate medical practice, patients typically
experience a sense of having colluded in their mistreatment, or
they fear that they have colluded or will be accused of having
colluded. Then they tend to feel guilty for being so angry.

The generation of DES daughters, versed in women's rights
and generally more comfortable with aggressive feelings than
their mothers are, tend to see the DES story in terms of doctors'
paternalism toward women who were socialized to be too compliant and agreeable. Some of the daughters decide to be unlike
their mothers in this respect; they become vigorously and
usefully assertive about their own health needs and care.

A twenty-eight-year-old DES daughter was alarmed to learn of
her mother's passivity and compliance during pregnancies in
which DES was prescribed. Determined to inform herself and
become an active participant in her own maternity experience,
she studied and discussed conception and pregnancy with her
husband for several years before they decided it was time to

have a child. Perhaps for reasons related to DES, this woman had trouble conceiving and as a result had numerous procedures that she could not have anticipated. Her sorrow at infertility was compounded by her frustration at becoming dependent on physicians, even to the point of taking hormonal fertility medication, thus repeating the experience of her mother that she had tried so hard to avoid.

This woman attempted to use her mother's passivity as a corrective for her own behavior but did not repudiate the entire system of care when she could use it for her benefit.[6]

Other daughters are so eager not to repeat what they perceive as their mothers' passivity and victimization that they go to the opposite extreme, either avoiding doctors, to their own detriment, or presenting themselves to physicians in a hostile and aggressive manner that precludes the development of any positive relationship. This stance masks the same passive needs during illness as the mothers' more overt passivity.

A DES daughter who believed passionately that women should inform themselves about and care for their own bodies went for all her medical care to a women's health center, where physicians were employed only on an occasional consultative basis.

At age twenty-four, she began to lose weight and felt a tumor developing in her pelvis, for which her friends urged her to seek medical attention. She delayed and rationalized for several months, hoping that the tumor would go away. Then, in panic, she chose from the telephone book the first gynecologist who could give her an immediate appointment. She saw him for a consultation. Fortunately this physician, chosen at random, turned out to be extremely competent. He operated immediately, on the basis of the history and his examination, and called a psychiatrist in, anticipating that his diagnosis of ovarian carcinoma would be traumatic for this young woman.

He had not had any time to develop a relationship with the patient. He experienced her as hostile and demanding, and he expected that she might become profoundly depressed. He himself became sad, even tearful, when he spoke to the psychiatrist about the approaching death of such a healthy, active woman. The operation he performed was total organ removal plus attempts to remove scattered cancer tissue.

A massive and aggressive chemotherapy regime was instituted immediately following surgery. When the psychiatrist visited the patient, he was startled to find a frail, balding, calm woman hugging a gigantic Teddy bear. The patient reported with surprising resignation that she was going along with all the recommended treatments and had every expectation of resuming work and of being able to marry as planned the following year. Her only expressed concern was that she might not be able to have children.

Denial was her way, at this point in time, of coping with the overwhelming trauma. And she had no more interest in developing a relationship with the psychiatrist than she had with the surgeon.

Because of her long-standing refusal to acknowledge any value in physicians, this woman had no opportunity to develop a way to deal with them, so that when her dependency on doctors broke through her defenses, she expressed it in an infantile fashion. Her devaluation of all physicians had led her to choose at random, on the assumption that one would be as good (or as bad) as another. She thus precluded any possibility of a collaborative relationship with a carefully chosen doctor. Unable to relate to physicians, whom she inevitably associated with DES, she finally developed a relationship with a nurse in the oncology clinic with whom she discussed the problems of selecting stylish wigs and getting along with her boyfriend.

Because of the solid personal basis of the physician-patient tie, it is usually only the most extreme situations that will mobilize general outrage against doctors. Medical malpractice suits reflect such outrage. Usually they stem from situations in which the patient was totally passive, as in the case of surgical errors witnessed by others while the patient was asleep, errors that are grievous in impact and grossly visible. Yet there is a reluctance on the part of most mentally stable patients to complain publicly about their personal physicians.

To date, all but one of the lawsuits involving DES mothers and daughters have been brought against the pharmaceutical companies that manufactured the drug. The exception is a suit against the University of Chicago (Mink et al. 1982), in which the mother-plaintiffs claimed that they did not know they were taking DES in the original Dieckmann studies. These patients had not had a long-standing personal relationship with their physicians; they had come to a university clinic for routine prenatal care of their first pregnancies and, they allege, were given what they were told were "vitamin pills." Thus, they claim, they were merely unknowing participants in an experiment. The significant factor here is that these women had no sense of having colluded with the doctors who gave them DES. They sued the institution that provided their care—so far, a unique instance.

DES families and the general community as well have expressed sustained anger at the inadequacy of attempts of physicians to contact DES mothers to alert them to risks and to their offspring's need for medical surveillance. Most DES-affected individuals, however, initially experienced anger at their physicians only transiently and then quickly rationalized it away. They focused on all the good the doctors had done for them—not at all surprising when the physician had helped them produce a baby. Angry feelings toward others are easily dissipated by feelings of gratitude and loyalty. The mothers indeed became angry at themselves and experienced guilt for feeling ungrateful and disloyal, and this attitude has tended to discourage active and useful protest.

There are, of course, realistic and human limitations to medical practice. Slippage inevitably occurs between what is known or believed and what is done. Even where the basic rule of medical care, "primum non nocere," has been breached, it is difficult for sensible people, doctors and patients alike, to say with certainty that the practice is a bad one and should cease. People prefer to rationalize the criticism, to make excuses, to blame third parties or themselves, or to empathize with the doctor's error in order to

avoid a confrontation that would disrupt the doctor-patient relationship. The human bonds and psychological complexities of
the doctor-patient relationship insulate and protect this powerful
attachment.

7

The Doctors' Dilemma

*Medicine is the most distinguished of all the arts, but
through the ignorance of those who practice it, and
of those who casually judge such practitioners, it is
now of all the arts by far the least esteemed.*
— Hippocrates, *The Law*

*I will use treatment to help the sick according to my
ability and judgment, but never with a view to injury
and wrong-doing.*
— Hippocrates, *The Oath*

Doctors prescribed DES for thirty years in a regimen they believed would prevent and treat reproductive failures. This prescription was motivated, as we have seen, by the wish to heal and
to rescue. In a single therapeutic gesture the doctor could integrate his desires to heal, nurture, and create with his rescuing,
grandiose, and heroic impulses. But the medical art, twenty-five
centuries after Hippocrates, remains imperfect. DES, the drug
that promised to improve on nature and to create life, instead led
to anomalous physical conditions for many and death for a few.
And the implications of DES have been as serious for the medical
community as for its users. It has affected the doctors who gave it,
those who continue to care for DES patients, and those who are
now prescribing new drug regimens, confident—as were those

who originally prescribed DES—that these treatments are more beneficial than deleterious.

Unlike their patients, physicians seem to have responded to the aftereffects of DES with little overt guilt or self-blame. Relatively few obstetricians have complied with requests from their own professional organization, the American College of Obstetrics and Gynecology (ACOG) that they actively attempt to contact exposed female offspring in order to provide needed information and examination.[1] Indeed, the failure of private physicians to reach DES daughters has been responsible for the development of public health outreach programs in several states which provide clinical screening for daughters and referral centers for sons, as well as education and consultation services for physicians (Glebatis and Janerich 1981). The National Cancer Institute has compiled DES information for physicians and patients in the form of free pamphlets. These have been distributed widely, but it is not possible to determine whether the doctors use them.[2] We do know that most DES patients have learned about their situation though public health efforts and the mass media rather than from their prescribing doctors. The responses of many physicians to such public intervention into their private domain have ranged from indifference to resentment to active disapproval.

The apparent underreaction of physicians to DES is puzzling and distressing and not adequately explained by their fear of lawsuits. Patients repeatedly report feeling more upset by their physicians' nonchalance than by the fact of the DES exposure itself. It seems to us, however, that this nonchalance actually masks a range of complex defensive reactions.

At a staff meeting of obstetricians and gynecologists, we presented various patient responses to DES and discussed clinical approaches to DES daughters who require continued obstetric-gynecologic observation. In the discussion that followed, an older obstetrician stated that he himself had never given DES to any of his patients, although he knew that many other doctors in town had prescribed the drug; he now felt satisfied that he had been right and his colleagues wrong. With that comment he left the meeting. A second physician in the older age group admitted that he had prescribed DES on several occasions, but only when the patients insisted; it was, he recalled, the time of the Korean War, and several of his patients, eager for the pregnancy to succeed, had heard of DES and pushed him into prescribing. He, too, then left the meeting. Another older gynecologist said that since there was now a formal protocol, follow-up care for the daughters, and the original cancer scare had been overestimated, there was no longer any cause for alarm. The audience relaxed. Finally a young staff physician pointed out that in the old days people didn't know about adequate drug trials, and, of course, nothing like DES would ever be given by his generation. There was some sparring between the generations of physicians present. Then the remaining older practitioners left to return to their private offices.

The first physician proclaims innocence, then departs. The second blames the patients, rationalizes, and also leaves. They do not wish to be identified with the community of doctors who erred; nor do they want to learn how to treat the DES-exposed or to hear any more about the problem. The third denies that a problem exists. The young physician reassures himself that it couldn't happen to his group. And most of the physicians, whether prescribers of DES or not, flee the scene of discussion.

The DES experience addresses the deepest fears of doctors: the fear of facing their own mistakes; of failing in the eyes of peers and younger colleagues; of being criticized, regulated, and even sued. Further, it elicits feelings of powerlessness and helplessness in the face of uncertainty and chronic, unremitting illness, often in young people from families painfully reminiscent of their own. (Many doctors insisted that their wives take DES.) Finally, we believe that the DES experience stirs unconscious and universal fears of sadism, maiming, and castration. The contrast between the original promise of DES, to create life, and its actual devastating effects suggests an explanation for the subdued, even paralyzed, responses of practicing physicians in the terms we applied to the responses of patients—in terms, that is, of trauma.

The DES story is a paradigm of the doctor's personal and professional struggles. It has often been presented as an example of what the powerful and mostly male medical profession has done to women. In our view, this is an insufficient account. To see it merely in male/female terms oversimplifies and clouds our understanding of a complex human event.

Let us begin with medical training. Doctors are trained to diagnose and treat illness. But they are peculiarly unprepared to cope with iatrogenic illness—with those medical problems that arise from the activity of physicians themselves.[3] Faced with iatrogenic illness, the doctor's image of himself as a healer of the sick is inverted: he becomes the cause rather than the cure of illness. Most doctors go out of their way to avoid concluding that a patient's problem has been iatrogenically induced.

Since the spectre of incompetence cannot be tolerated in modern medicine, it may be easier for doctors to rationalize and disregard error than face up to it. Scientific medicine is accustomed to treatment regimens that are used for a while, then fall into disfavor and are replaced. Whatever their shortcomings regarding the admission of errors, doctors are accustomed to failed efforts, and to tragedies and death.

There are crucial experiences in training and early practice that make it more possible to tolerate mistakes, to learn and grow from them.[4] All beginning professionals make mistakes; that is why they need some modulating protection from excessive guilt, which could lead to an emotional withdrawal from patients and a reluctance to take necessary risks. Patients may perceive this cautious stance as indifference on the part of the doctor. On the other hand, without such modulating protection, doctors may develop another stance, one that seems to the patient to be like the previous one but is actually quite different. If doctors have no defenses against the consequences of their own mistakes, they may develop a rationalizing, seemingly cavalier "we all make mistakes" attitude, which allows them to deny their actual feelings of responsibility. This suppression of their own feelings seems also to limit their responsiveness to the feelings of their patients. They may come increasingly to regard the patients in detached, even formulaic ways—in the service of maintaining their self-esteem, which depends on their being exemplars of competence.[5]

Their emotional unwillingness to confront errors has contributed to the failure of many of the physicians involved with DES to participate in efforts to identify and locate DES-exposed people. Some doctors argue that casefinding is not a reasonable use of their time or funds. Others oppose it because of their fear of exposing their mistakes and of resulting lawsuits. Some argue that casefinding creates problems: it is logistically difficult; it may generate great anxiety in those contacted; it may "iatrogenically" produce excessive bodily concerns. Alarmist media coverage, they claim, and perhaps with some truth, may drive away as many people as it locates. Nonetheless, we believe that casefinding is a necessary part of responsible contemporary medical practice.

Leslie J. DeGroot, professor of radiology and medicine at the University of Chicago, was pivotal in mobilizing casefinding— "recall programs"—for individuals radiated in childhood and vulnerable to thyroid carcinoma. This was probably the first major instance of large-scale casefinding in modern medicine.[6] Dr. DeGroot recalls:

> I felt responsibility had to be taken. . . . Resistance was pretty strong. . . . Records were not available. Doctors didn't answer. Just wouldn't. Hospitals were afraid of exposure. . . . Publicity was effective. *Time* and *Newsweek* articles prompted people to phone. . . . Even specialists were reluctant to support recall programs. Some felt recall was more dangerous than letting the tumors develop fully and then operating. The incidence of death from these tumors is very low. I don't agree with them. . . . It was the lawsuits against various hospitals that spurred the recall programs. Most of them are hospital based, not hospital initiated. Private practitioners didn't look. The kids don't know. Only their parents. If they can remember. . . .
>
> Radiation was not used at the U of C very much. . . . You know, it did some good. People would have lost their hearing from chronic *otitis media* [ear infections]. It was the days before

antibiotics. . . . It's more complicated with DES because there is real uncertainty whether DES was effective at all. . . .

There was a theory that extensive enlargement of the thymus caused suffocation in babies. For example, 10,000 kids from Rochester, New York, had their thymuses radiated, and one doctor followed those 10,000 kids. Some hospitals irradiated every newborn as they left the nursery—they called this technique "the ray of sunshine. . . ."

Now there is a wave of parathyroid tumors beginning, in relation to the original group of irradiated thyroids, producing hyperparathyroidism. . . .

It's easier for us academic endocrinologists than for the private ob-gyn practitioners. For DES the ones who gave it are the ones who have to casefind. For us it's one generation of doctors who gave the radiation and another generation who are engaged in casefinding. And the treatment is definitively repudiated. It was all over by 1952. . . .

It's clear the lawsuits stimulated the casefinding for thyroid cancer. As to DES, there the need to casefind is so clear because the tumors are so dangerous, and the earlier the discovery, the better the prognosis. . . . It's hard for ob-gyns to deal with this. Until recently, it's been a specialty filled with old-wives' tales. . . . For thyroid, there was an argument about relative danger from the surgery versus the risk of the tumor. That won't hold for DES. But to do recall programs, you need lawsuits or pressure from citizens' groups. . . . You know, these days the time between scientific discovery and "usual and customary practice" is very short.

Many physicians are able to affirm in their professional lives the grandiose fantasies that led to their choice of medicine as a profession. They surround themselves with a coterie of adoring patients and admiring colleagues and family who maintain their sense of specialness. They are often kindly individuals who go to considerable lengths to take care of their patients, thus enhancing and protecting their own feelings of nobility.

An obstetrician who prescribed DES for twenty years was well informed about the risks of DES exposure. With some arrogance, he stated that he had no need to inform his patients of any harmful effects of DES since they knew that he had given them their babies and were eternally grateful to him. There was no need for him to waste his money on a casefinding project. He said that it was more "convenient" for him not to think about the problem at all, except to reassure the occasional worried patient who approached him. He was not worried about lawsuits. He had, he said, the best malpractice insurance around.

It is ironic that such patronizing behavior may actually help these unrealistic "supermen" to be effective doctors. There are situations that only physicians who are grandiose to the point of megalomania will dare to tackle—often to the patient's considerable benefit. In appreciation for accepting such challenges, however, these physicians may unreasonably demand unswerving and infinite loyalty. As long as the patient cooperates and complies with all the doctor's orders, the doctor will take care of everything and will not abandon the patient. If the physician's behavior, opinion, or authority is questioned in any way, however, he is apt to feel injured and to become furious with the patient. His sense of authority often extends even to patients' families.[7] A doctor with such an approach may, of course, be just right for some patients, especially at certain times. The problem is that this kind of treatment fosters blind loyalty in the patient at the same time that it affirms the infallibility of the physician, leaving neither prepared for the crisis of an error.

There is another kind of doctor with the opposite problem, one who can become demoralized, self-blaming, and ineffectual in response to his own mistakes.

An elderly, depressed man jumped in front of a train in a suicide attempt and lost a leg. His young physician berated himself for having given the patient leave from the psychiatric hospital. He went to see him on the orthopedic ward, apologizing over and over, saying it was all his fault. His behavior became a burden to the patient. The doctor could not separate his own feelings from those of the patient and no longer acted as his physician but as a grieving friend. He had difficulty attending to his other patients and taking responsibility for their care.

Physicians are trained to deal with external catastrophe. But as individuals, they are no less vulnerable to the inner pain of catastrophe than other people are. In fact, studies show that many physicians have experienced intense vulnerability or illness in childhood (Deckert 1976). This personal experience of vulnerability combined with professional training for coping with catastrophe still does not prepare physicians sufficiently to deal with medical error. On the contrary, the combination of personal background and formal training may do just the opposite by decreasing the physician's capacity to empathize with patients in crisis. If the doctor is defending against recognition of his own feelings, medical training may provide him with the means to avoid empathizing with the patient, to deny the human side of a trauma and instead focus sharply and narrowly on the mechanical and technical aspects of the problem.

It may seem paradoxical that a physician who can accept his own helplessness in the face of trauma is in the best position to help a patient, because only such a physician can allow and even encourage the patient to be active. The doctor who insists on being the only active participant in the relationship, however, on doing *to* the patient rather than *with*, forces the patient into a passive and helpless position that can make him more childlike, anxious, and angry. By contrast, a physician who empathizes with the patient's wish to be brave and endure suffering can more effectively enlist the patient's collaboration in the treatment.

The training of physicians tends to deal with the anxiety that is ever present in the care of the sick by excessively distancing the doctor from the patient. Most students entering medical school are open to the human experiences they will encounter and eager to encounter them. But many feel overwhelmed by "too much too soon." One student reported that he had wanted to be a pediatrician but found that he "felt too much" for the babies and young parents he saw on the pediatric service. He decided to go into a less emotionally draining field. He felt ashamed of being "so mushy." Had he received sympathetic support for his pained responses to his patients' suffering and supervision to help him deal with distraught parents, he might have become a fine pediatrician.

The gradual process by which a young medical student learns to respond professionally to his patients without losing his capacity to empathize with their feelings requires that he accept his own limitations as a doctor. This is a quiet but crucial aspect of an ideal medical training. The student will learn this if his teachers can display a tolerance for helplessness, passivity, and vulnerability in themselves and others and a willingness to admit feelings of concern in the face of loss and death. This capacity reflects the unheroic, conserving dimensions of medical care. And it is this ongoing, caring medical practice that DES offspring need in particular. Yet despite the value of this type of medical care, it is nevertheless the heroic measures that are the high points of medical training, medical practice, and medical history. The moments in which the doctor is a hero—the quick apprehension of a diagnosis, the photographic recall of the latest developments as reported in the most prestigious journals, the rapid transformation of a critical medical problem into a biologically sound technical solution—these are charged with the exhilarating and prized grandiosity of the physician's role.[8]

It is not difficult to see how entertaining such ambitions can lead to premature and uncritical enthusiasm about a drug like DES or to widespread use of a medicine that promises rescue from having to stand by helplessly while nature takes its sometimes cruel course during pregnancy. The values expressed by these heroic images help us understand why many obstetrician-gynecologists do not seem to comprehend the experience of those exposed to DES. To the gynecologist, most DES daughters have routine, uninteresting, technically simple problems—if the problems are defined in narrow biomedical terms. Nothing to get excited about, not what gets the doctors exhilarated.

The primary continuing care of people with chronic problems, like those of the DES-exposed, in fact constitutes a great part of medical practice. The maintenance and care of such patients require a kind of comforting and supportive presence that nurses have traditionally been trained to provide. Physicians, by contrast, are trained in a more active mode: the way they strive for diagnosis and cure challenges illness rather than yields to or works with it. How much the doctor can permit himself or herself to be a quiet caretaker, one who brings comfort and maintains health, is the issue. Health professionals need to be able to do both. The caring capacity of physicians invariably stems from deep-rooted personal qualities they had long before medical school, for their training encourages the development of aggressive, assertive behavior.

As we have said, the powerful impulse to help, to save, and to transform has always been a force within medicine. This concern to heal has two major aspects—an innovative and active one, and a conserving, attending, more passive one. Modern medicine, with its crucial reliance on extreme technical competence and its close links to biological research and constant discovery, strongly emphasizes the active, innovative aspect. There is a widespread conventional notion within the profession that the tender, humane, caring dimension of medicine is a feminine characteristic and should perhaps be left to the nurses. It has even been suggested recently that the quality of caring will be enhanced in the medical profession as a whole as increasing numbers of women continue to enter all branches of medicine.[9] An important question to follow over time, however, will be whether the increasing numbers of women do indeed bring more "feminine" values and styles of relating to medicine or whether the women develop "masculine" values and take on the biomedical mentality and norms of the work world they enter. In general, women tend to be more open to their own vulnerability, to have been patients themselves more frequently, and to be more easily empathic with patients (Apfel 1982). We think, however, that the relation between the innovative and conserving aspects of medicine is not quite so simple.[10] The socially defined "female" function can be satisfied just as well by a man as by a woman; it should be a valued dimension of every physician.

An obstetrician-gynecologist left his position at a distinguished teaching hospital to become chief at a large community hospital in another part of the country. His dream was to set up a new department of obstetrics and gynecology. The day the news came that the new program was certified, the physician was radiant. He was overheard saying to a colleague, "Now, from the very first day, I can show the new residents that women are human beings." Intrigued, we tracked him down. He explained that, in his opinion, most residency training programs focused excessively on the necessary and important surgical techniques and equipment for patient care at the expense of attending to the whole patient. "Childbirth is only an entree to her total care. That is why I so much want to teach the residents that they can never lose sight of the larger context."

We have been dealing in this chapter with some responses of physicians to DES that stem from natural tendencies we all share to some extent but that seem to be supported, if not exacerbated, by the very character of modern medicine. Our discussion thus far has focused on the behavior of individual physicians; we now turn our attention to the character of obstetrics-gynecology as a medical specialty and to the collective behavior of doctors as members of an organized profession.

Obstetrics-gynecology is the "happy specialty." It is classified as a surgical specialty and requires surgical training and a surgical mentality, marked by assertive, decisive behavior. Yet, unlike most surgery, it also involves long-term personal relationships with its all-female clientele, relationships that frequently extend far beyond the term of pregnancy and include the routine care of healthy patients. The culminating drama of birth at which the obstetrician presides is appealing and rewarding. The fantasy among doctors about obstetrics is that the physician will get to know patients who are healthy, attractive, young, cooperative, and grateful. Obstetricians say that they chose their field to make people happy by giving them babies. They tend not to like people who are sick and sad.

Yet many of the patients seen by the obstetrician-gynecologist are not happy, not fertile, and have chronic, unremitting, incurable problems. Patients cannot always be rescued from their ailments, and the doctor may be deeply frustrated by the failure of his practice to match his original fantasy.

Surgical specialties including obstetrics and gynecology have a value orientation toward strength and activity, much more than, say, family practice, primary care, internal medicine, or psychiatry does. Medical students choose their specialties on the basis of many conscious factors—monetary rewards, demands on time, public and professional prestige, intellectual challenge, the amount of information to be mastered, the requisite skills, personality fit, medical school experiences on specialty rotations, geographic location, length of residency training, opportunity to exercise medical responsibility. (Becker et al. 1961; Lyden et al. 1968). The choice of specialty also involves unconscious factors, commonly centering around the young doctor's comfort or discomfort with his own aggressive impulses.

Underlying all specialty choices lies the general motivation for pursuing a medical career—the wish to help and serve. This is never a pure and unalloyed feeling, however. Anger, aggression, and hostility are present—unconsciously and, at times, even consciously—here as in all human experience. A measure of growth and maturation is the use to which these negative but normal feelings are put and how they are converted to acceptable forms. They are never totally eliminated.

The role of the physician and the problems with which doctors deal touch upon deep universal fears. The fear of doing harm, even killing, and, conversely, of being vulnerable, even losing a sense of integration and wholeness—all these fears can be heightened in physicians by their power and skill, as well as by their empathy with patients. One of the mechanisms by which physicians cope with these fears is by participating in the flow of life, especially in birth, which is symbolically restorative. The healing power of medicine is balm to these fears in the physician as well as in the patient.

During the years of medical school, students develop a professional self-image (Huntington 1957). They think of themselves increasingly as doctors with each patient contact and gradually move away from identifying primarily with the patient. In the course of their ordinary activities, doctors must inflict pain "in the patient's best interest," whether in the form of surgery, side effects of drugs, diagnostic procedures, or even psychotherapeutic interpretations. The doctor cannot, and optimally should not, feel the pain the patient feels. Doctors who are seen as insensitive or unfeeling by patients may be just doing their jobs; however, they may also go to the extreme of denying that the patients are suffering.

A jovial and renowned obstetrician attended a clinical research talk on the emotional stress of pregnancy. Data were presented from interviews with pregnant women and their husbands to show that pregnancy is a time of great anxiety about malformation, mutilation, and death. Normal pregnancy was experienced by many of the interviewees as physically uncomfortable, emotionally stressful, and a time of conflict in close relationships. The obstetrician objected strenuously to the presentation, saying that he had been working with pregnant women for twenty-five years and he knew for certain that pregnancy is a time of personal bliss and fulfillment with no conflict—except for a very few highly neurotic individuals.

This physician denied all doubt, fear, ambivalence, and conflict in patients he considered to be normal pregnant women. He staunchly maintained the fantasy that he was a jolly Santa Claus delivering babies to contented couples.

More complex responses to patients present more anxiety for the physician.

A young obstetrician who looked particularly haggard confided that she had been awake for the previous three nights attending a patient with uterine hemorrhaging. The patient had multiple medical problems, including a problem with blood coagulation. She had lost two previous children and hoped to have a child. The doctor had been apprehensive about whether conservative, watchful waiting and fluid re-

placement would work; she had consulted with older colleagues and decided to wait and see. She was relieved that her
treatment had saved the patient's life and preserved her uterus
and reproductive capacity.

This doctor had not arranged the usual sharing of responsibilities for her patient with her colleagues because she knew
that if her peers had charge of the case they would have performed a hysterectomy several days earlier rather than sit out
the anxiety and treat the bleeding more conservatively. She was
upset by a request that the case be presented at the weekly
"maternal morbidity and mortality review" because she feared
the censure of her colleagues for the risk she had taken in
waiting, even though the outcome for the patient had been
favorable. She believed that other doctors would have preferred the risk of operating on someone with a bleeding problem in order to get it over with to the risk she had taken by
waiting.

This physician felt torn between her identity with her professional group and her responsibility to her patient. She acted on
the patient's behalf but feared that she would be criticized by her
colleagues. She found support among the older, more experienced doctors in her department. As a woman, she was sensitized
to her patient's feelings; as a person, she was able to tolerate
anxiety over time. Her wish to maintain not only the patient's life
but her capacity to produce life was enhanced by her personal
experience. For three days, she felt more involved with her patient than with her colleagues. When the patient improved, the
doctor's anxiety shifted from illness and prognosis to "what will
the other doctors say?" She acted bravely in her conservative
approach, but had the patient died she would have been a villain,
and she feared retribution for having taken too risky and heroic a
measure. By making an independent medical decision, the doctor paid the price of the additional anxiety that comes from turn-
ing counter to one's peer group.

In private, physicians tend to be very competitive and to crit-
icize one another's treatment of patients. In public, however, they

rarely confront other doctors with inappropriate behavior. Within the medical profession, self-policing takes place alongside self-protection and group preservation. It has been very difficult to have open public discussion among doctors about the issues involving DES. Physicians are not at ease debating issues around "usual and customary practice." Where treatment involves one doctor, one patient, one technique, the medical community does well in self-observation and the upholding of standards. Where complex policy issues and third-party involvements are concerned—such as relations to the pharmaceutical and insurance industries, the public policies determining health care delivery, the government regulators—physicians are far less able to perform with the high quality that characterizes individual practice. The model of medical education is "See one, do one, teach one." There is little in medical training that prepares physicians to grasp and debate the policy issues that now shape the profession.

When Dieckmann presented his studies in 1953 showing the ineffectiveness of DES in a general prenatal practice, much of the subsequent discussion at the meeting of the American College of Obstetrics and Gynecology centered on personal loyalties rather than on scientific merit. One of the gynecologists present said, "As a former Bostonian, I would be entirely lacking in civic loyalty if I had not used stilbestrol [DES] in my private practice" (Dieckmann et al. 1953, p. 1080).

Sociologists have studied the patterns of diffusion of new practices throughout the medical profession (Greer 1977). Coleman and his associates (1957) showed that doctors who work in hospitals and medical schools and who are more oriented toward the opinions of other physicians will use a new drug before their colleagues in the community who are more oriented toward their patients. In each group, however, there is what they call a "snowball" effect, a chain reaction of increasing acceptance and use. Professional and personal connections establish who uses which drug. The momentum increases over time, and use increases despite diminishing validation of the new technique. This was the DES experience.

Use and availability of medications are also related to affluence, social class, and expectations (Duff and Hollingshead 1968; Mahler 1977). DES was given primarily to middle-class, urban, white patients who wanted the newest and the best.

A professional woman in her mid-fifties recalled that at thirty-two, she had had two miscarriages and was receiving gynecologic care through a health insurance program in New York City. Her physician was a well-regarded obstetrician-gynecologist who maintained a private practice as well. One of her friends, with no history of problem pregnancy, was a private patient of this very same doctor. She learned many years later that this friend had been given DES, while she had not.

Given the prestige of medical research, the diffusion of new techniques and drugs begins mainly in university hospitals. This process, when it works, is rapid and effective. It quickly becomes socially acceptable to use new drugs and socially unacceptable not to do so. With DES, the whole profession went awry. The DES case is an example of the inadequacies of research and communication, and of institutional *hubris* and the failure of regulation within the profession and the community.

For most physicians, loyalty to the group and to tradition can act to encourage further growth and personal courage, not only maintenance of self-esteem and occasionally self-deception. It is surprising how often a physician has in his office or library pictures of heroes or idealized teachers or the legendary historical figures in his or her specialty. They function as reminders to the doctor of the highest standards of the field. A positive force for continuing medical education is the competition to produce excellence that would satisfy one's heroes, that measures up to the best one's profession has achieved, and that permits one to share the results of the work with colleagues in open professional encounters. These positive standards act not just as inspirations to do better but as constraints to limit poor medical practice. Thus the elitism of medicine works to set and maintain standards and create group coherence. It also works to exclude deviants, to disseminate new treatments prematurely, and to distance patients. The competitiveness, aggression, and perseverance required to become a physician, the intelligence and interpersonal skills, can all be detriments or assets to modern medical practice. Group loyalty among physicians, while frequently functioning to inhibit full honesty and courage and creativity, can also help to ensure ethical conformity and high standards.

The sense of belonging to an elite group can be a source of strength that helps the individual physician tolerate and accept error and responsibility, or it can merely provide escape and promote denial and self-aggrandizement. Physicians who deviate from or contradict accepted practice may be severely criticized, even extruded from the medical community.

The doctor who does confront an error may be regarded as an enemy of his group rather than a hero. A famous example from a century ago poignantly illustrates this:

> Ignaz Philipp Semmelweis, a Viennese obstetrician, noted in 1847 that the death rates of mothers after delivering babies were highest in those clinics where the students came to the obstetrical wards from lectures on pathology or from the dissecting room. He prescribed that all those entering the wards must wash their hands carefully. The mortality rate of patients on his service diminished immediately and greatly, while mothers continued to die at high rates on all the other services. Despite this evidence, and despite his affirmation that the cause of puerperal (post-delivery) fever could be found in blood poisoning, he was attacked by all the great obstetricians of Vienna. His only support came from a few distinguished nonobstetrical physicians. He was forced to resign from his position at the Vienna Krankenhaus and moved to Budapest, where he published a great work on asepsis in obstetrics, a work which eventually led to a new era in his field. His persecution by his colleagues contributed to a nervous breakdown; he died at age forty-seven in an insane asylum. In 1894 a monument was erected to him—in Budapest.[11]

Semmelweis made a major discovery that saved countless lives. He died a tragic martyr to unyielding traditional norms and customs. Handwashing—with the implicit assumption that physicians could be unclean—was not a readily accepted practice. Then, as now, physicians preferred complex procedures to simple prophylactic ones.

After the well-controlled studies of DES in the 1950s, its usage declined somewhat, but it did not cease until the association with cancer was discovered in 1971. By then, other treatments had been developed for high-risk pregnancy, and the reaction of doctors to the loss of the DES regimen was primarily resentment of government interference in medical practice.

Indeed, the magical quality of the sex hormones that captivated medical attention in the 1920s and 1930s is still with us, sustaining the desire to create life and to preserve youth and health. A 1981 textbook of gynecology and obstetrics (Romney et al.) suggests that DES be used as the treatment of choice for abnormal cervical mucus. If the mucus is too thick, DES will change it to the "normal watery kind" that permits sperm to get through and enhances fertility; if there is too little cervical mucus, DES will increase the production of secretion from the endocervical canal, which may also enhance sperm transport.

Physicians currently treat infertility problems with a variety of techniques, including the prescription of hormonal agents such as clomiphene and human menopausal gonadotropins to aid conception or of beta-mimetic drugs to maintain a shaky pregnancy. These are accepted practices. Whatever anxiety there may be about replicating the DES experience in the future is well hidden by the enthusiasm for these drugs that can help bring forth babies in the present. The future and potential hazards of using hormones in pregnancy are not so impressive or powerful as something that works in the here and now. And the fact that other colleagues are using such drugs with some success will be enough to spread the practice and to make it seem that refusing to prescribe hormones is unwarranted—even if a physician simply wishes to withhold usage until more results are in, perhaps with the DES experience in mind.[12]

Because physicians are still responding in the same old way to the dilemma of choosing between future hazards and present victories, history may well be repeating itself. Doctors' persistent tendencies to minimize the impact of DES may be a sign of defensive maneuvers against this distressing possibility. Many obstetrician-gynecologists who prescribed the drug still believe that it worked in high-risk pregnancies and that history will prove them right.[13] Findings of decreased reproductive capacity in DES offspring have repeatedly been attributed to inheritance from mothers with fertility problems despite good studies linking the problem to DES, not heredity. More epidemiologists, pathologists, and psychiatrists than gynecologists have demonstrated concern about DES in the aftermath.

Burnham (1982) has documented the shift within the twentieth century from medicine's "golden age," about 1900–60, when doctors were most highly esteemed, especially in the post-war period coinciding with DES usage, to the current view of physicians and the profession in general as cold, costly, and uncaring. The DES experience parallels and probably contributed to this trend.

From beginning to end—from the invention of the drug through experimental application, widespread usage, suspicions of ineffectiveness, discovery of the true effects, and the half-hearted denying response of the profession to the final long-term chronic treatment of the victims—DES has truly been a paradigm of modern medicine, displaying its best and worst. If the story is a sad one, it is nevertheless instructive—but only if all of us, doctors and patients, individuals and the community, can bear to hear it told.

8
Final Reflections—What Next?

The story we have told is a somber one. We have tried to describe the events attending the use of DES without either muckraking, on the one hand, or denying their seriousness, on the other. Our objective has been to learn from the experience. DES is not the only scandal in modern medicine, perhaps not even the worst. And though much has changed in the practice and structure of medicine in the past forty years, the likelihood of another iatrogenic disaster of similar proportions is still with us. It is to this likelihood and the reasonable hope that we can avoid or limit it that these concluding remarks are directed.

Many of the recent changes in the policies and institutional structures of medicine are clear improvements and may help to prevent another DES-like disaster. The development of informed consent, the elaborate procedures for conducting randomized clinical trials, the emergence of public-interest investigative groups, the improvement in medical reporting by the popular media, and the growth of an informed public of medical consumers all may lessen the probability that the more egregious mistakes of the DES story will be repeated.

On the other hand, there are many problems inherent in these very developments to which all of us, within and outside the medical profession, need to become sensitive. The policy of informed consent is obviously good, and yet, as many observers have noted, it has severe limitations. Desperate, frightened, or even habitually compliant people will frequently give their "informed" consent to the use of a drug or procedure that they might question in other circumstances. As we have argued, the very role of patient diminishes a person's independent judgment and lessens the meaning of informed consent. But beyond this general situation, the major consequences of taking DES did not appear for fifteen to twenty years, and then mainly in the offspring, not in the patients. Who can give informed consent for events whose consequences are twenty years in the future and primarily affect someone else?[1]

The development of sophisticated and carefully controlled randomized clinical tests is subject to the same problems. Who spends twenty years conducting an experiment before collecting and publishing the data? The enormous growth of the medical research establishment, supported and promoted by the government, the public, the drug industry, and the academic medical profession, has accelerated and systematized the development of new drugs and medical technology. At the same time, the very size of this medical research establishment has inevitably created a new special-interest group with its own needs and concerns. The great improvement in reporting medical developments in the mass media frequently means that a much better informed public demands access to new or experimental procedures before they are adequately tested or understood (Rourk et al. 1981). The public-interest investigative groups, by their very success in exposing to public scrutiny the improprieties and malfeasances of some contemporary medical practice, may also serve to undercut the public confidence that an effective health-delivery system needs from its clientele.[2]

On balance, of course, all these developments are for the good. It is not our intention here to offer concrete policies or programs that might be suggested by the DES experience. Many other commentators have made such proposals, and they and others will continue to do so. We obviously support ongoing public discussion and debate on these matters. There needs to be constant public discussion both of general policy and of specific issues and developments; the pros and cons of, for example, heart transplants, dialysis, and recombinant DNA need to be thoroughly

aired both within the medical establishment and in the public at
large. But so do the general procedures of the FDA in approving
new drugs, the allocation of federal funds to various areas of
medical research, and the content and structure of the curricu-
lum in medical schools.

Such ongoing dialogue is extremely valuable, even necessary,
for the health of modern medicine, but in our opinion it is not
sufficient. DES, after all, was extensively discussed from the
1930s until its approval by the FDA in 1941. But the participants
in the dialogue were largely unaware of the degree to which their
positions were governed by their special interests, the prevailing
fashion, and their passions. There is no reason to think that the
participants in contemporary and future debates will necessarily
be any different. As long as that is the case, the tragedy of DES
may recur, always in a new guise, and always to the shock and
dismay of the actors in the drama.

In this connection, it is well to remember that there actually
were in the 1950s several well-designed controlled clinical trials
of the effectiveness of DES in high-risk pregnancies. These studies indicated that DES was simply ineffective. Admittedly, the
samples were small, and thus the results were inconclusive. Nevertheless, it is remarkable that these studies were almost totally
ignored in the enthusiasm of the medical establishment and the
general public to bring DES into wide use. If the system had
worked the way it was supposed to, these early, small-scale studies
would have served to stimulate the large-scale, conclusive studies
that should have been, but never were, done. Of what use are
excellent, refined formal procedures if no one pays attention to
their findings?

New technical developments and improved institutional ar-
rangements will not get at the problem of the continual recur-
rence of iatrogenic disaster. What is needed, rather, is a shift in
the character of the participants. We already have an abundance
of technical virtuosity and theoretical sophistication. Now we require a special kind of human excellence or, to use an old-fash-
ioned word, virtue. In antiquity, Aristotle called it prudence, or
Practical Wisdom; in the eighteenth century, Kant called it judg-

ment; in the early twentieth century, Alfred North Whitehead called it foresight. But whatever name it goes by, it refers to a developed human capacity to make independent, autonomous judgments about urgent practical matters for which there are no general rules.

In respect to this capacity, modern medicine may face its most striking dilemma. Most of the enormous power of contemporary medicine derives from the extraordinary interplay between its technical capacities and its theoretical understanding. There is a synergy between these two in that new technical developments make greater scientific understanding possible, and scientific understanding frequently leads to the creation of new techniques. In its fascination with these twin sources of its power, medicine is in danger of forgetting that our understanding is and will always remain profoundly limited and that our technical abilities are always subject to profound misuse and error.

Take DES, for example. In their zeal to demonstrate its effectiveness, researchers steadily increased the size of the dosages until they were giving single doses that far exceeded a woman's lifetime production of estrogen. It is technically feasible to give such dosages, of course, and the results may well enhance scientific understanding; but surely prudence suggests that the experimenter should approach such dosages only with extreme caution and the most careful preparation. Prudence focuses not only on what we know and can do but also on what we do not know and cannot do. We need to remember our ignorance and our clumsiness as well as our knowledge and our skill. We need to be aware of our zeal for truth and for healing, not only as sources of power, but as passions that can lead to self-deception and errors of judgment. And, of course, the consuming public, both as individual patients and as the politically organized community, needs in its way to exercise the same moderation and prudence in the demands it makes on the medical profession. Such reflections as these can easily become platitudinous, but it is well to remember that the DES disaster derived precisely from the passion for truth and the desire to improve the quality of life.

The story of DES, for all its modernity, bears many of the

marks of classical tragedy. Everyone acted in good faith, with the best of intentions, and within the established norms of medical procedures of the day. Thus the consequences seem unavoidable. What we can learn from the story is not who to blame or what technical procedure we can employ to avoid the errors of our predecessors, but that we are subject to the same stresses and temptations as the actors in the DES tragedy. The story is a sad one, but it need not be futile if we can learn from it. In the words of Aeschylus, "From suffering comes wisdom."

Notes

Introduction

1 Dr. Burke may be contacted at the Department of Obstetrics and Gynecology, Beth Israel Hospital, 330 Brookline Avenue, Boston, Mass. 02215. The address of the Massachusetts branch of DES Action is P.O. Box 126, Stoughton, Mass. 02072. The headquarters of DES Action National can provide the addresses of other local chapters. On the East Coast, it is based at Long Island Jewish–Hillside Medical Center, New Hyde Park, N.Y. 11040; on the West Coast, at 1638B Haight Street, San Francisco, Calif. 94117.

2 Anke A. Ehrhardt, Ph.D., and Heino F. L. Meyer-Bahlburg, Dr. rer. nat., may be contacted about work in progress at the Program of Developmental Psychoendocrinology, New York State Psychiatric Institute, Columbia University, 722 West 168th Street, New York, N.Y. 10032.

Chapter 1

1 Allen, Danforth, and Doisy (1939, pp. 466–68) cite Iscovesco (1911) in the French literature, Fellner (1912–13) and Hermann (1915) in the German literature, and Frank and Rosenbloom (1915) in the English literature for their work on finding estrogenic activity in ovarian extracts. Injecting ovarian extract reversed the uterine atrophy which occurred after ovaries were removed surgically, or in natural menopause. Normal nonpregnant rats, mice, and rabbits were used to test for estrus induction after their own ovaries had been surgically removed.

2 Aschheim and Zondek's work is cited by Dodds (1932) as one of the better outcomes of the research on sex hormones. An accurate, rapid diagnosis of pregnancy was established that was used for forty years. The urine of a pregnant woman was injected into an immature female mouse; the mouse was killed forty-eight hours later, and its ovaries showed premature maturation of the

ovarian follicle. The "oestrin" in urine later turned out to be luteinizing hormone.

3 DES-type drugs that may have been prescribed to pregnant women include the following:

Benzestrol	Estrosyn	Palestrol
Chlorotrianisene	Fonatol	Restrol
Comestrol	Gynben	Stil-Rol
Cyren A.	Gyneben	Stilbal
Cyren B.	Hexestrol	Stilbestrol
DES	Hexoestrol	Stilbestronate
DesPlex	Hi-Bestrol	Stilbetin
Dibestil	Menocrin	Stilbinol
Diestryl	Meprane	Stilboestroform
Dienestrol	Mestilbol	Stilboestrol
Dienoestrol	Methallenestril	Stilboestrol DP.
Diethylstilbestrol	Microest	Stilestrate
Dipalmitate	Mikarol	Stilpalmitate
Diethylstilbestrol	Mikarol forti	Stilphostrol
Diphosphate	Milestrol	Stilronate
Diethylstilbestrol	Monomestrol	Stilrone
Dipropionate	Neo-Oestranol I	Stils
Dithylstilbenediol	Neo-Oestranol II	Synestrin
Digestil	Nulabort	Synestrol
Domestrol	Oestrogenine	Synthoestrin
Estilben	Oestromenin	Tace
Estrobene	Oestromon	Vallestril
Estrobene DP.	Orestol	Willestrol
	Pabestrol D.	

Nonsteroidal estrogen-androgen combinations include:

Amperone	
Di-Erone	Teserene
Estan	Tylandril
Metystil	Tylosterone

A nonsteroidal estrogen-progesterone combination is Progravidium.
Vaginal cream-suppositories with nonsteroidal estrogens are AVC cream with Dienestrol and Dienestrol cream. (NCI—NIH publication no. 81–2049, Appendix A, p. 19.)

4 Shimkin and Grady (1940) thus confirmed the earlier work of Loeb (1935), Lacassagne's finding on mice (1938), and Geschickter's observations on the rat (1939).

5 A forty-year-old male chef manifested mysterious breast development, a decrease in facial hair, and a voice that was becoming higher in pitch. There was no internal estrogen source to account for his rapid feminization—no tumor or liver disease. He casually asked his doctor whether his unusual diet might account for his symptoms. He then revealed that for the previous six months he had been trying to save money by eating chicken necks discarded by his restaurant. When a sample of the chicken necks was analyzed, DES pellets were discovered.

In Puerto Rico and Italy a current epidemic of thelarche—precocious puberty, or stunted growth with early sexual development in boys under ten and girls under nine—has been correlated with high chicken consumption. The FDA, the U.S. Department of Agriculture, the Center for Disease Control, and an independent investigator at the University of Pennsylvania have been unable to reach consensus as to the presence of high estrogen levels in chicken samples (see *Ms.* 12, December 1983).

6 Dr. Wise Burroughs of Iowa State University wrote in *Science* (July 1954) about a method of including DES in cattle feed that did not involve inserting DES pellets. Thus the food additive could still provide advantages to the producer without, it was thought, endangering the consumer. Burroughs patented this method in 1956. Orenberg (1981, p. 135) reports that Burroughs' patent generated over $3 million.

7 Feedlot owners went to the federal courts in 1973 to try to block FDA bans on DES additives and pellets in beef. Beef meat, especially liver and kidneys, continued to show substantial amounts of DES—even more when analytic methodology was improved. The FDA collected additional evidence of infractions and moved for a final ban on 1 November 1979. Orenberg (1981, p. 136) states that "so strong was the siren call of extra profits from super-fat, DES-boosted cattle" that illicit use continued; by 1980, the FDA had prosecuted 115 feedlot owners for giving their cattle DES after the 1979 ban. The experience in Puerto Rico, though inconclusive, suggests that infractions may still occur.

8 Bell 1980, p. 164. Prior to the 1930s the distinction between propriety/patent products and ethical/prescription products was blurred by the fact that most ethical drug companies produced a line of patent drugs and sold them in chain drugstores, pharmacies, and department stores without prescription. Eli Lilly was the one exception, distributing materials only through physicians. Ethical drugs have exceeded proprietary ones in sales only since World War II, a time of phenomenal growth for the drug industry. For further discussions on drug regulation in the United States, see Temin 1980, Wade 1972, and Young 1967.

9 The first joint drug application was filed for sulfathiazole in 1939, when four companies banded together to expedite a review of 700 cases in order to get the life-saving sulfa approved.

10 The twelve drug companies were Abbott Laboratories; Armour Laboratories; Ayerst, McKenna & Harrison; George A. Breon & Co., Inc.; Charles E. Frosst

& Co.; Eli Lilly & Co.; Merck & Co., Inc.; Sharp & Dohme, Inc.; E. R. Squibb & Sons; The Upjohn Co.; Winthrop Chemical Co.; and John Wyeth & Bro., Inc. Parke-Davis was initially involved as well but dropped out before the joint application was filed.

11 Bell 1980, pp. 38–39. D. E. Shorr, S. H. Geist, and U. J. Salmon were the first to question FDA approval. They were joined by the fourth dissenter, Raphael Kurzrok, in 1940.

12 The following editorial appeared in *JAMA* 113 (1939): 2323–2324:

ESTROGEN THERAPY—A WARNING

The last ten years has seen a remarkable development in our knowledge of the endocrines. Especially great strides have been made in the therapeutic application of sex hormones, notably the estrogenic substances. Pure highly potent preparations of estrogens are being manufactured. Furthermore, biochemists are constantly striving to discover new compounds of even greater activity or to increase the efficiency of those already known. Pharmaceutic chemists are looking for better preparations which may be protected by patent. Much attention has been given to the preparation of estrogens for oral use, since the advantages of such therapy over hypodermic administration are appreciable.

Two new compounds—ethinyl estradiol and diethylstilbestrol—have been used clinically in recent months and have been shown to be as effective as the injected estrogens in moderate doses. General acceptance of these compounds has been prevented by complaints of disagreeable symptoms following their ingestion. Ethinyl estradiol induced in a considerable percentage of patients nausea, vomiting, headache, and malaise. Diethylstilbestrol, however, has been prescribed, especially in England. The reports as to the toxic reactions of this substance are quite conflicting, some investigators stating that gastric distress is the only complaint, that this is experienced by from 5 to 10 per cent of the patients, and that it vanishes after a few days of administration. Others have found side reactions in greater numbers. One group of American investigators has observed as high as 80 per cent of the patients exhibiting untoward reactions, including cutaneous eruptions, psychosis, lassitude and liver damage. Apparently a thorough investigation of this compound is in order before it can be prescribed for routine therapy. In this issue of THE JOURNAL (p. 2312) will be found a statement of the Council on Pharmacy and Chemistry on the present status of stilbestrol; also three articles published under its auspices.

The conflicts in the reports on these substances and the opinions of some authorities on the possible harm from estrogen therapy should warn against long continued and indiscriminate therapeutic use of estrogens. Like numerous other therapeutic agents estrogens are effective under the proper circumstances, but there may be definite danger when they are used unscientifically. In this connection the possibility of carcinoma induced by estrogens cannot be ignored. The long continued administration of these proliferating agents to patients with a predisposition to cancer may be hazardous. The idea that estrogens are related in their activity only to sex organs should be abandoned. Other tissues of the body may react in an undesirable manner when the doses are excessive and over too long a period. This point should be firmly established, since it appears likely that in the future the medical profession may be importuned to prescribe to patients large doses of high potency estrogens, such as stilbestrol, because of the ease of administration of these preparations. (Copyright 1939, American Medical Association; reprinted with permission)

13 The total exchange of information involved in the approval of the 25 mg pill was as follows: Eli Lilly and Co. filed a supplementary New Drug Application in April 1947. They submitted a photostat of a paper by White and Hunt (1943) which reported 181 cases of threatened toxemia in diabetic women. They alluded to a paper by Smith and Smith (1946), cited Karnaky (1942) on 86 cases, and quoted verbal confirmation of Karnaky by Abarbanel. The FDA first responded by conferring with "outstanding experts in the fields of obstetrics and endocrinology" that "your recommendation for the use of the drug in toxemia of pregnancy is too broad and inconclusive" (26 May 1947 letter from Ernest Q. King, acting medical director). Lilly produced further documentation from Smith and Smith about their regime and their findings of decreased toxemia and prematurity and increased fetal survival in cases treated with DES. Approval was then granted on 27 August 1947 (letter from W. J. Rice, Director of Chemical Control).

14 As published in the 1953 *Physicians' Desk Reference* (*PDR*), Smith and Smith advised the following regime for oral administration of DES:

Week of pregnancy dating from first day of last menstrual period*	Daily dose
7th & 8th	5 mg
9th & 10th	10 mg
11th & 12th	15 mg
13th & 14th	20 mg
15th	25 mg
16th	30 mg
17th	35 mg
18th	40 mg
19th	45 mg
20th	50 mg
21st	55 mg
22nd	60 mg
23rd	65 mg
24th	70 mg

25th	75 mg
26th	80 mg
27th	85 mg
28th	90 mg
29th	95 mg
30th	100 mg
31st	105 mg
32nd	110 mg
33rd	115 mg
34th	120 mg
35th	125 mg

*Subtract 2 weeks to obtain age of embryonic fetal life.

15 The seven papers were Smith and Smith 1954; Gitman and Koplowitz 1950; Davis and Fugo 1950; Ross 1953; Pena 1954; Plate 1954; and White, Koshy, and Duckers 1953. The last group studied diabetes.

16 King in 1953 reviewed more than twenty reports of treatments of threatened abortion. He found large groups of patients, from 1,000 to 24,289, who had been treated with stilbestrol in small to huge doses, other estrogens, progesterone in small and large doses, vitamin E, wheat germ oil, and thyroid (usually with vitamin E or progesterone). The rate of miscarriage or spontaneous abortion increased with each previous pregnancy loss. Of 2,792 women without previous miscarriage, 67 percent carried to term regardless of the kind of treatment they received; of 1,820 who had two or more previous miscarriages, 61 percent did well regardless of the nature of treatment. These rates are significantly higher than placebo response, or the 33 percent of patients who do well with any treatment, however inert the pill may be.

Care and attention and a belief in the prescribed treatment by both the prescribing clinician and the patient affect the pregnancy outcome in a positive and significant manner.

Miscarriage results from a multiplicity of incompletely understood psychological, neurological, and endocrinological factors. Mann (1959) chose patients who had three or more previous miscarriages and found that the majority could carry to term with psychotherapy. His study shows the value of dealing directly with the anxiety and apprehension created by a history of pregnancy loss.

A recent reference on the often underestimated emotional sequellae of pregnancy loss is Friedman and Gradstein 1982. In papers directed to obstetricians and gynecologists, Seibel and Graves (1980) and Seibel and Taymor (1982) address the emotional impact of miscarriage. Additional work documenting the value of medical attention to high-risk pregnancy is reported in Clifford 1964 and Jacobson and Reid 1964. Fortney and Whitehorn (1983) report on a new index that attempts to unify and quantify the definition of high-risk pregnancy.

17 The seven controlled trials were Crowder, Bills, and Broadbent 1950; Robinson and Shettles 1952; Ferguson 1953; Dieckmann et al. 1953; Randall et al. 1955; Reid 1955; and Swyer and Law 1954.

18 Comparison groups can be selected in various ways. The best is a random sample in which each member of the total population studied has an equal chance of receiving the treatment, as if those who received DES were names picked at random from a hat. Alternate controls are chosen more systematically and with a greater potential for bias; for instance, every other woman entering a clinic receives DES and the alternate woman receives an inert pill. Simultaneous controls are a contrived group similar in most respects to the treatment group and treated concurrently but not necessarily drawn from the same population pool (see MacMahon, Pugh, and Ipsen 1960, pp. 239–43). Historical controls, of the sort used by Smith and Smith, compare the current treatment group to a group treated previously at a different time and place.

19 Brackbill and Berendes (1978) reviewed the Dieckmann paper and concluded that it provided enough evidence to conclude that DES was dangerous as well as ineffective.

20 The *PDR* has been published annually since 1947 by Medical Economics Company, Inc., with the cooperation of the drug manufacturers. The listings in the PDR are the same as the package inserts provided with each drug. The Smith and Smith dosages "used to prevent accidents of pregnancy" were listed every year until 1962. Then, between 1962 and 1968, "pregnancy accidents" were included as an indication for DES but without the dosage schedule. In 1969 a warning appeared: "Because of possible adverse reaction on the fetus, the risk of estrogen therapy should be weighed against the possible benefits when diethylstilbestrol is considered for use in a known pregnancy" (p. 819). In 1973 the pregnancy use was contraindicated.

21 Edwin P. Jordan, editor of the 1958 edition of the *Modern Drug Encyclopedia and Therapeutic Index,* was at that time a lecturer in social and environmental medicine at the University of Virginia Medical School. He does not mention any use for DES in pregnancy although in that same year the PDR provided the whole treatment plan.

22 Heinonen (1973) and the Boston Collaborative Drug Surveillance Program examined data on DES use in 51,000 pregnancies in twelve hospitals between 1959 and 1965. On the basis of these data they estimated that more than 100,000 mothers per year received the drug between 1960 and 1970. Epidemiologists believe that this estimate is high. Continuing surveillance of estrogen-usage patterns for epidemiological purposes is reported in Rosenberg et al. 1979.

23 In 1970 three reports of cases in young females appeared in the scientific literature: Herbst, Green, and Ulfelder; Herbst and Scully; and Droegemuller, Makowski, and Taylor.

24 We spoke with Dr. Olive Smith just prior to her death at age 81 in March 1983. Dr. Smith and her husband never lost their conviction that DES had been a

valuable treatment for the toxemia of pregnancy because it improved the placental circulation. She said that investigations continue to this day to document her original contention and referred us to Dr. Nicholas S. Assali, professor of obstetrics and gynecology at UCLA. Dr. Assali responded warmly, "It is about time that people from the Mecca of Science have decided to tell the truth . . . work on the placental production of progesterone with the administration of estrogens has been completed as a Ph.D. thesis from one of my trainees from Brazil, Dr. Marcelo Zugaib. . . . It is 88 pages, well written, if you can understand Portuguese." The Zugaib thesis confirms the Smith hypothesis, but it does not go further to document the validity and efficacy of using DES in human pregnancy.

25 Dr. Emmanuel Friedman, Professor of Obstetrics and Gynecology, Harvard Medical School, personal communication, November 1982.

26 Canario, Houston, and Smith (1953) published a follow-up comparison of three- to five-year-olds who had been born prematurely. The forty-one children whose mothers took DES were, on the average, heavier at birth than the fifty-eight whose mothers had received no hormone. By ages three to five, the groups were alike in most ways.

27 DES in high dosages—50 mg a day for three to five days—can inhibit implantation and thus prevent pregnancy from unprotected intercourse within the previous twenty-four hours. As of 1983, according to Roger Eastep, supervising consumer safety officer, Division of Metabolism and Endocrine Drugs, FDA, no NDA has ever been approved for the use of DES as a postcoital contraceptive (personal communication, 7 November 1983).

28 DES is currently used in infertility cases where cervical mucus is inadequate. Hormonal drugs are also used to induce ovulation. Clomiphene citrate (one brand is Clomid), a drug that is given orally, works in about 70 percent of cases. Human menopausal gonadotropin (HMG), or menotropins (Pergonal), contains follicle-stimulating and luteinizing hormones and is given by injection to stimulate the development of follicles and the maturation of ova. These ova can be harvested via laparoscopy for *in vitro* fertilization. The HMG material is extracted from human menopausal urine. Hyperstimulation and multiple pregnancy are known side effects of both Clomid and Pergonal. These hormones can also induce changes in the developing fetus.

A nonhormonal and nonestrogenic drug used for inducing ovulation is bromocryptine mesylate (Parlodel). This inhibits prolactin secretion, thus suppressing lactation and sometimes restoring fertility. The dangers, if any, of fetal exposure to bromocryptine are not yet known.

Chapter 2

1 Silverman 1980a, table 10-2, "Results of some 'Proclaimed' Therapies in the Development of Perinatal Medicine," p. 85, and the discussion of detergent mist treatment following the table. Also see Silverman 1980b.

2 Bell (1984) has studied DES as a case example in the development of medical technology. Other examples are numerous: e.g., Banta 1979, on fetal monitors; Chalmers 1974; Silverman 1980a, 1980b, and 1980c.

3 The United States has attempted in recent decades to develop more independent research organizations, such as the congressional Office of Technology Assessment and the Institute for Medicine. The National Institutes of Health have elaborate ties to academic medicine, and, as we have seen, the FDA has connections with both the drug industry and academia.

4 Between 1939 and the early 1950s numerous articles appeared in the medical literature linking tonsillectomy and poliomyelitis, especially of the bulbar type (see, for example, Krill and Toomey 1941, Aycock 1942, and Pederson 1947). Francis et al. 1942 highlighted this dangerous association in their report of the experience of the "K" family of Akron, Ohio. Of the six children in the "K" family, five were tonsillectomized on August 22. By September 7 all five had bulbar poliomyelitis; three of the children later died of this disease. The one child who was not operated on showed no sign of illness although the polio virus was recovered from his stool.

   A retrospective view on tonsillectomy by Haggerty (1968) concludes that the original justification for the operation—to prevent streptoccocal infections and rheumatic fever—has been disproven. Tonsillectomy should definitely not be performed when the risk of polio is high. Because of the development of effective anti-polio vaccines in the 1960s and the widespread inoculation of infants, polio epidemics are no longer prevalent.

5 Veith (1965) traces the history of hysteria from Ancient Egypt to Charcot and twentieth-century psychoanalysis. Simon (1978, p. 238) relates the wandering uterus concept to interpersonal relations in ancient Greece.

6 Bassuk (1983) discusses ovarian surgery as a widespread treatment of insanity in the late nineteenth century. References from that time document the conviction that castration was a valuable treatment for mental illness. (See Wells, Hegar, and Battey 1886; Clark 1888; Barnes 1890; and Tyrone's 1952 review of late nineteenth-century gynecologic practice.) Although Freud (1911) discussed Schreber's paranoia about castration as if it were completely delusional, the use of sadistic restraining devices in Schreber's childhood has been documented by psychoanalyst William Niederland (1974). Schreber's doctor, Flechsig, had promoted castration as a treatment for insanity.

   Spitz (1952) describes clitoridectomy as a treatment for masturbation. A journal was published on the subject from 1892 until 1923. On 15 November 1981 the *Washington Post* carried an article about the current use of DES to inhibit masturbation in the mentally retarded.

   Celia Bertin, in her 1982 biography of Marie Bonaparte, describes a procedure for operating on the external female genitals to enable orgasmic pleasure (pp. 140–41). Genital-mutilative surgery is still practiced on women throughout the world, perhaps with the same basis in fantasy but with the expressed purpose of improving marriageability and decreasing sexual desire (see Thiam 1983). Nonpathological conditions in women continue to be made into medical problems; see Love, Gelman, and Silen 1982.

7 Hysterectomy statistics have been compiled by the Centers for Disease Control and are summarized in a report on premenopausal U.S. women aged fifteen to forty-four. (U.S. Department of Health and Human Services, April 1981).

8 Dysfunctional vaginas as a result of vaginectomy are reported in Seaman and Seaman 1978. Some scarring and vaginal shortening were described in the article by Sherman et al. 1974. Gynecologist Allen Berlin, one of the original Detroit group performing partial vaginectomies, commented on the atmosphere of high anxiety about the connection between adenosis and cancer in the early 1970s. He acknowledged the problem of post-operative vaginal dysfunction in some cases (personal communication, 8 March 1984).

Chapter 3

1 The National Cancer Institute of the National Institutes of Health (NIH) has operated a DES information office since 1974 which has answered thousands of inquiries and mounted many public and professional educational campaigns. Write to Department DES, NCI, Office of Cancer Communications, Building 31, Room 10A19, Bethesda, Md. 20205, or call Alice Hamm at (301) 496–6641. (See the bibliography under National Cancer Institute for a list of NCI publications.) This office also makes available reprints from the National Cooperative Diethylstilbestrol Adenosis Project (DESAD), which gathers data according to unified protocols at five major medical centers: Massachusetts General Hospital, Boston, Mass.; Mayo Clinic, Rochester, Minn.; Baylor College of Medicine, Houston, Tex.; University of Southern California, Los Angeles, Calif.; and Gunderson Clinic, LaCrosse, Wisc. A list of publications of the Registry for Research on Hormonal Transplacental Carcinogenesis (see note 7 below) and other DES-related references is available from the NCI office.

2 John-Gunnar Forsberg's tissue culture research (in Herbst and Bern 1981) suggests that DES works chemically to influence the formation of superficial cells by the underlying stroma, or tissue. He has shown how chemical variation in the fundamental tissues can induce an unexpected type of epithelial cell.

3 Forsberg and Kalland (in Herbst and Bern 1981, p. 20) summarize biochemical studies. They state that alpha-fetoprotein, a glycoprotein present in relatively high concentrations in fetal and neonatal plasma, differentially binds (and thereby deactivates) different estrogens. In the rat and mouse, alpha-fetoprotein binds steroidal estrogens, but little DES and no hexestrol. Human alpha-fetoprotein does not appear to bind natural or synthetic estrogens. However, human fetal tissues have a general and substantial capacity for sulfation and inactivation of all biologically active estrogens. This mechanism in the fetus exceeds the maternal capacity to deactivate estrogens but is

still incomplete, to judge from estrogenic effects on the developing urogenital tract. There is some evidence that estrogenic effects may be cumulative and that early exposure sensitizes the organism. See Banbury Report no. 8 (1981) and Shapiro and Slone 1979.

4   Meltzer (in Herbst and Bern 1981, p. 164) suggests several mechanisms for the carcinogenicity of DES: (1) DES undergoes oxidative and conjugative metabolism in humans to produce reactive metabolites that are capable of damaging DNA, thus initiating tumors and promoting cell growth; (2) DES has a mitogenic effect specifically on estrogen target organs; estrogen receptors may accumulate the reactive metabolites and even facilitate their access to nuclear DNA; (3) DES metabolites may be preferentially formed in estrogen target tissues by particular enzymes. Peroxidase is one enzyme that can activate DES to DNA-binding metabolites and is present in tissues that depend on estrogens for growth.

5   Canario, Houston, and Smith (1953) addressed the question of DES-induced malformations in children exposed in utero. They compared 42 DES and 60 control children at age two to three-and-a-half years and found no increased incidence of congenital malformations in those exposed to DES. "This and the other foregoing evidence of harmlessness of stilbestrol to the human fetus deserve emphasis because of the well-known toxic effect of estrogens upon the fetuses of rodents" (p. 1303). They go on to cite a 1942 symposium showing that small doses of DES in pregnant rodents produced abortion or resorption of the pregnancy and resulted in a high incidence of sex inversion in offspring carried to term. The malformations caused by DES in humans did not show up until the offspring reached puberty, years past the time frame of Canario et al.'s follow-up study. Speaking to this point, George Smith commented, "Who could predict thirty years ago that anything like this would develop? I mean regardless of the rat and mouse work" (quoted in Seaman and Seaman 1978, p. 14).

6   McLachlan, Newbold, and Bullock (1980) showed that 25 percent of mice given DES at the time of maximum reproductive organogenesis, in a dosage schedule similar to what Smith and Smith recommended for humans, developed epidermoid tumors of the vagina. One had vaginal adenocarcinoma (not clear cell type). There was also a low incidence of other tumors—benign leiomyoma and papilloma, and malignant stromal cell sarcoma and leiomyosarcoma. Three of these were located in the ovaries. The tumor incidence was dose-related, and 35 percent of the tumors were genital in location: vagina, cervix, and uterus. Newbold and McLachlan (1981) expanded the work on benign vaginal adenosis and adenocarcinoma in mice exposed to DES transplacentally.

   Pathologist Dr. Stanley Robboy (personal communication, November 1983) cites the work referred to above and that of Jones and Tacillas-Verjan (1979). The latter researchers found that mice given ovarian steroids developed tumors of the müllerian system, including adenocarcinoma of the vagina and cervix; these adenocarcinomas, however, were not of the clear cell type seen in human DES-exposed females.

7 The Registry for Research on Hormonal Transplacental Carcinogenesis, established in 1971 and supported by grants from NCI, records all cases of clear cell adenocarcinoma of the vagina and cervix occurring in women born in 1940 or later, whether or not there is a history of maternal hormone ingestion. Also, it studies all cases of genital cancer (vulva, vagina, cervix, endometrium, tube, or ovary) in any female born after 1940 with a reasonable possibility of exposure in utero to any exogenous hormone. It has actively sought referrals from all hospital obstetrics and gynecology departments and cancer specialty hospitals. Cases are evaluated clinically by Dr. Arthur L. Herbst of the Department of Obstetrics and Gynecology, University of Chicago, and pathologically by Dr. Robert E. Scully, Massachusetts General Hospital. See Herbst and Bern 1981, pp. 63–70, for discussion of the epidemiological findings from the Registry. For information, call Dr. Herbst or Dr. Marian Hubby at (312) 962–6671 or Dr. Scully at (617) 726–3956.

To date, cases of clear cell adenocarcinoma have been reported from almost everywhere in the United States, from South America, and from Europe. It is noteworthy that no cases are registered from Denmark or Finland, the two countries in which DES was never used in pregnancy. In about two-thirds of the cases there is documented maternal ingestion of DES or a related compound, ranging from 131 to 21,400 mg of the drug. The risk is increased by early exposure in utero; where DES was taken after the seventeenth week of gestation, there are very few cases of CCA and there is decreased adenosis. With increasingly early detection, survival rates at five years after diagnosis of CCA are now 80 percent.

8 Adenosis associated with in utero stilbestrol exposure was first described in the literature by Herbst, Kurman, and Scully in 1972. Since then, numerous gynecologists at many medical centers have described adenosis in DES daughters. The adenosis appearance of the cervix has become a pathognomonic sign pointing to a history of DES exposure before birth. See Lanier et al. 1973; Pomerance 1973; Vooijs and Wentz 1973; Stafl et al. 1974; Burke et al. 1974; Sherman et al. 1974; Robboy, Scully, and Herbst 1975; Morrow and Townsend 1975; Stafl 1975; Sandberg 1976; and Robboy et al. 1976.

9 Cervical erosion is a condition in which the area around the central opening to the uterus appears raspberry red in color; columnar instead of squamous epithelial cells cover the area and produce the red color. Eversion or ectropion means that the inside lining epithelium of the uterus is on the outside of the cervix. For drawings of these lesions, see Sandberg 1976. For photographs, see Herbst and Bern 1981 and National Cancer Institute 1981.

10 Burke, Antonioli, and Friedman 1981 and Ng et al. 1977 have now demonstrated that adenosis does not usually require treatment. Noller et al. reported in 1983 on the DESAD project which followed over 450 women for three years according to a strict protocol. They found that 53 percent showed no change

in that time span, 29 percent definitely improved spontaneously, and almost 7 percent seemed worse, though there was no malignant change. They too conclude that watchful waiting is the treatment of choice. In 1974 Sherman et al. had recommended wide excision of the areas of adenosis, performing a partial vaginectomy (see chapter 2, note 8). Schmidt et al. (1980) cauterized adenosis areas in the vagina and cervix. Cryosurgery, or freezing, and periodic "weeding" by punch biopsies (see Richart 1980) have also been recommended. Acidification seems to accelerate squamous metaplasia, according to Fowler and Edelman (1978). Herbst et al. (1974) used local progesterone intravaginally to expedite the transformation of adenosis. In 1976 Schmitt moderated a panel discussion of colposcopists who treated adenosis. The DESAD collaborative project recognizes vaginal adenosis coexisting over time with squamous metaplasia on colposcopic and histologic examination; these researchers use the term "vaginal epithelial changes" (VEC) to include both conditions.

11 J. G. Forsberg wrote his thesis in 1963 at the University of Lund, Sweden, on the controversy over how the vagina may develop from three different sets of epithelia—müllerian, wolffian, and urogenital sinus. He has since become a primary investigator of the embryology of the genital tract in humans and rodents. See Herbst and Bern 1981, pp. 4–25. Cunha (1976) is cited for his work on the developing urogenital tract. Prins et al. (1976) review the data on the embryogenesis of the vagina and discuss Forsberg's work; they postulate that prenatal estrogens accelerate differentiation of the vagina and uterus, cause male fetal müllerian ducts to persist, and prevent transformation of columnar epithelium to the squamous form.

12 For excellent technical discussions of sexual differentiation in utero, see Haseltine and Ohno, "Mechanisms of Gonadal Differentiation," and Wilson, George, and Griffin, "The Hormonal Control of Sexual Development," both in the 20 March 1981 issue of *Science,* edited by F. Naftolin, pp. 1272–1284.

13 Kaufman et al. (1977) first described the T-shaped uterus on hysterosalpingograms of DES daughters. Since then, correlations with pregnancy outcomes have been attempted. See Kaufman et al. (1980). Although there is an increased frequency of unfavorable pregnancy outcomes in DES-exposed daughters who have abnormal hysterosalpingograms, there is controversy about the statistical significance of these findings.

14 Dr. Ann Barnes of Massachusetts General Hospital had reported on menstrual patterns of DES-exposed daughters in 1979. Then in 1980 she used data from the DESAD project to compare the fertility experiences of a large pooled sample of DES and non-DES daughters. See Barnes et al. 1980.

15 Many authors and clinicians have addressed the subfertility problem. Besides Berger and Goldstein (1980), series of cases have been published by Rennell (1979), Cousins et al. (1980), Rosenfeld and Bronson (1980), Schmidt et al. (1980), Nunley and Kitchin (1979), Veridiano and Delke (1980), Stillman (1982), and Vessey et al. (1983). Depending on definitions and methodology,

the likelihood that DES daughters will have more fertility problems than nonexposed women ranges from 50 percent to zero. The general consensus is that a DES daughter is statistically about 35 percent less likely than a non–DES-exposed woman of equivalent age and health to have a noneventful pregnancy.

It is important to note that fertility rates refer to couples. The male partner is responsible for 40 percent of infertility problems. Age is also an important factor; female fertility is known to decrease with age from the early twenties. (Personal communication, Dr. Isaac Schiff, 14 December 1983.) For a discussion of age and fertility, see DeCherney and Berkowitz 1982.

New techniques such as in vitro fertilization are becoming options for infertile couples.

16 National Cancer Institute publication no. 81–2049 contains recommendations, based on the DESAD study, with photographic instructions for routine screening examinations and referral. Colposcopic photos are included.

17 Controversy exists about whether DES daughters are at actual risk of future cancer and have cause for concern. Interpretation of findings to date is being debated in the literature. Stafl and Mattingly (1974) and later Ng et al. (1977) expressed concern that the dysplasia seen in DES-exposed women would become invasive squamous cell carcinoma. Robboy et al. (1978, 1981) have compiled data from the DESAD project participants and note a lower incidence of dysplasia itself. They propose other causes for dysplasia besides DES-exposure—for example, the level of sexual activity and the fact that the DESAD populations are drawn from major medical centers, which receive high numbers of referrals. An eloquent and succinct statement of the squamous cell neoplasia controversy is found in Robboy et al. 1977. Routine Pap smears screen for squamous cell changes and are the best preventive measure.

18 See Banbury Report no. 8, a 1981 Cold Spring Harbor symposium on hormones and breast cancer. The epidemiology of breast cancer is presented along with discussions showing variable interpretations of the data.

19 Brian et al. (1980) found 8 cases of breast cancer in the 408 DES-exposed mothers compared to the expected 8.1 cases for the same number of nonexposed women in that locale.

20 Bibbo et al. (1978) reported that 693 women who were exposed to a maximum of 12 grams of DES over a 15- to 20-week period during their pregnancies twenty-five years earlier had slightly more breast cancers than their non–DES-exposed counterparts; the tumors started at an earlier age, and more of the DES women had died from the cancer. The exposed group had 32 cases (4.6 percent) of breast cancer; the unexposed had 21 cases (3.1 percent). Twelve of the DES mothers and four of the unexposed had died of breast cancer by 1980

21 Hubby et al. (1981, pp. 120–28) report that 34 of the DES mothers developed breast cancer with 15 deaths as compared to 28 cases of the cancer and 6 deaths among the unexposed women.

22 Beral and Colwell (1980) followed 80 diabetic women who received stilbestrol

and ethisterone and compared them to 76 nondiabetic, non–hormone-treated women who were pregnant at the same time.

23 See Ryan's 1978 editorial following Bibbo et al. 1978. Pietras et al. (1978) discuss the role of enzyme cathepsin B_1 in the tumor potential of DES.

24 Hoover, Gray, and Fraumeni (1977) also speculate about DES and the added risk of ovarian cancer. Whitehead et al. (1981) discuss hormones and the postmenopausal endometrium.

25 See also Meyer-Bahlburg and Ehrhardt 1980; Meyer-Bahlburg 1978; Reinisch 1974; and Reinisch, Machoven, and Karow 1977. Hier (1982) has looked at spatial ability with decreased androgens. Dr. Norman Geschwind and his co-workers at the Beth Israel Hospital, Harvard Medical School, are studying handedness and neuroendocrine dysfunction in DES-exposed offspring with the cooperation of DES Action, Mass.

26 Vessey et al. (1983) traced records and sent questionnaires to the physicians of women who had received DES in a controlled trial in the 1950s. In a study comparable to the Dieckmann trials, Swyer and Law in 1954 had admitted 813 patients. In the Vessey follow-up 561 cases were sought and the general practitioners returned information on 93.9 percent. Thirty-nine of 259 DES-exposed women and only 20 of the 271 nonexposed—a highly significant difference—were reported to have psychiatric symptoms including depression, anxiety, childhood behavioral problems, schizophrenia, anorexia nervosa, mental retardation, epilepsy, addiction or alcoholism, personality defect, psychosocial problems, and phobic neurosis. This small study suggests connections that are not yet understood.

27 Bibbo et al. 1977. Even less conclusive results are reported in Herbst and Bern 1981, pp. 103–19. See also Yalom (1973) and Beral and Colwell (1981) for reports indicating a shift away from masculine, heterosexual behavior in DES-exposed sons. This has also been found in a small survey by Dr. Richard C. Pillard, psychiatrist at Boston University School of Medicine (personal communication, June 1980).

28 Henderson et al. (1979) have done a case-controlled study in Los Angeles; their results suggest that risk of cancer of the testis is increased by exposure to estrogen during the time of fetal differentiation. Conley et al. (1983) report on a testicular cancer, seminoma, in a DES son. Vessey et al. (1983) found one fetal teratoma of the testis in their DES follow-up group. Up-to-date information on reported cases is available from the Registry of Male Tumors Associated with DES, Tufts–New England Medical Center, 171 Harrison Avenue, Boston, Mass. Any new male tumor cases should be reported to this registry.

Chapter 4

1 The Vietnam veteran's chronic traumatic response may seem very distant from the DES experience, but consider the sense of anxiety and helplessness about the fertility and quality of life of future generations in the wake of Agent

Orange exposure. There is also a similarity in the ambiguous relationship between victim and alleged perpetrator.

According to Ray Scurfield, associate director for counseling at the Readjustment Counseling Service of the Veterans' Administration in Washington, D.C., 20 to 60 percent of Vietnam veterans exhibit life-threatening behaviors and pronounced delayed and chronic responses to stress which seem to be more prevalent than among veterans of other wars. This phenomenon is thought to be due to the guerilla nature of the war, the constant rotation of soldiers in and out of Vietnam, and the conflicted responses of the American public to the war. On the other hand, in previous wars there was no conception of post-traumatic stress disorder, so that if a veteran's response to trauma was prolonged, chronic, or recurrent, physicians gave it another diagnosis. Nonetheless, the chronic traumatic responses seem especially severe and widespread among Vietnam veterans. Both homicidal and suicidal behaviors are more pronounced, but no reliable national statistics are yet available. Dr. Scurfield is planning to launch a national incidence and prevalence study with Dr. Ray Blank (personal communication 8 November 1983). For excellent discussions of the post-Vietnam syndrome see Figley 1978, Friedman 1981, and Yesavage 1983.

2 Hackett, Cassem, and Wishnie (1968) did a study of 50 patients who had myocardial infarctions (heart attacks) and were cared for in a coronary intensive care unit. They classified 20 of these patients as "major deniers," people who expressed no fear during their hospital stay; 26 as "partial deniers," those who denied being frightened initially but at some point in their stay admitted feeling some fear; and 4 as "minimal deniers," patients who complained of anxiety and admitted being frightened. There was no relation between denial and the patients' moods; everyone reported depression, hostility, and agitation. Fifty percent of the deaths took place among the minimal deniers, although they constituted only 8 percent of the total sample. None of the major deniers died; further, they had fewer complications and left the hospital sooner. Elaboration of this research can be found in Froese, Vasquez, Cassem, and Hackett 1974; and Froese, Hackett, Cassem, and Silverberg 1974.

3 The pattern of response to rape was defined by Sutherland and Scherl (1970) and expanded by Burgess and Holmstrom (1979). Authors who have considered human reactions to trauma in the most extreme circumstances, such as the Holocaust and atomic explosions, include Warnes (1972), Kinston and Rosser (1974), Stern (1976), Lifton (1963), and Kijak and Funtowicz (1982).

4 Clinicians working with Holocaust survivors repeatedly notice the central importance of the survivors' development of affiliative bonds, whether in the camps, in hiding, or on the run. An especially moving elaboration is found in Levi 1959. For descriptions of the later somatic and psychological consequences of concentration camp internment, see Hoppe 1971; Eitinger and Strom 1973; and Eaton, Sigal, and Weinfeld 1982.

Chapter 5

1 Thoughtful commentaries on the primary maternal relationship can be found

in Bibring et al. 1961; Newton 1973; Friedl 1975; Hammer 1975; Friday 1977; Chodorow 1978; Cohler and Grunebaum 1981; and Ehrensaft 1980.

2 Comprehensive discussions of female adolescent development can be found in Sugar 1979; Kirkpatrick 1980; Notman and Nadelson 1978, vol. 1; and Nadelson and Notman 1982, vol. 2.

3 DES exposure, like other physical problems, can disrupt optimal growth and development. There is a growing body of literature in adolescent psychiatry on the problems of serious illness and its effects on adolescence. See Schowalter 1977, 1983a, and 1983b.

4 Other personal accounts of DES trauma can be found in Cook 1981; Fenichell and Charfoos 1982; Shopper 1980; and Sipe 1982. Schwartz and Stewart (1977) summarize clinical data from a DES program. Meyers (1983) tells the DES story with many personal histories. These accounts demonstrate how, as with other traumas, the reverberations of the DES experience continue for many years.

5 We can only speculate about the possible relationship between anorexia nervosa and DES; the subject merits further investigation. For an excellent review article on anorexia nervosa per se, see Maloney and Klykylo 1983.

6 Universal fantasies about the power of women are discussed in Lederer 1968 and Lerner 1974. For presentations of mythic forms and symbolism, see Weigert 1970 and Neumann 1963.

7 Historian Nancy Weiss (1977) has written an interesting comparison of these manuals of the 1950s and 1960s and the turn-of-the-century "infant care" manuals produced by the U.S. Children's Bureau. All of these manuals were filled with practical advice, but the tone of the government pamphlets was more matter-of-fact and solicitous of the mother.

8 Some mothers of DES daughters have attributed their daughters' failure to marry and apparent apathy about childbearing to DES exposure. This observation from several of our interviews cannot be presented as fact but might serve as a hypothesis in a study of the emotional sequellae of DES. Dr. Elaine Gutterman of New York's Mount Sinai Hospital has interviewed DES mothers and has demonstrated a continuing concern about their daughters' welfare and fertility. Part of her doctoral thesis was presented to the American Society of Psychosomatic Obstetrics and Gynecology in March 1983.

9 Fewer studies have been conducted of DES male offspring than of females, there are fewer investigators, and there have been less cooperation and follow-up involving males. For reports of work on DES sons, see Gill, Schumacher, and Bibbo 1976; Henderson, Benton, and Cosgrove 1976; Hoefnagel 1976; Bibbo et al. 1977; Cosgrove, Benton, and Henderson 1977; Mills and Bongiovanni 1978; Gill et al. 1979; Driscoll and Taylor 1980; and Conley et al. 1983.

10 There are individuals who are genetically male but appear to be anatomically female at birth; they are reared as females and have their femininity affirmed by appropriate parental attitudes and behavior. When such people reach adolescence and are discovered to have ambiguous genitals and to lack a

normal vagina and uterus, they wish for a vagina and a uterus, not for the male organs that may also be present in rudimentary form. With the exception of rare cases of hermaphroditism, involving a sexual hormone enzyme defect in genetic males that allows for prenatal androgen priming of the developing brain tissue but causes anatomic female genitals, the people studied want the organs that go with their assigned gender. This assumes normal parenting and does not apply to transsexuals who are clearly physiologically male or female but nevertheless desire to have the organs of their opposite anatomic gender. See Stoller 1979; Money and Ehrhardt 1972; and Money, Hampson, and Hampson 1957.

Chapter 6

1 Significant writing on this subject includes medical sociological studies of the experience of being a patient and personal accounts of that experience. Although they are beyond the scope of this book, the reader may be interested in Blackwell 1973; Bologh 1981; Byrne and Long 1976; Cousins 1982; Davis 1968; Fisher and Todd 1982; Francis, Korsch, and Morris 1969; Frankel 1980; Lazare, Eisenthal, and Wasserman 1975; Rabin 1982; and Ramsey 1970. For an excellent analysis of the doctor-patient relationship with which we are very much in tune, see A. Freud 1964. For a historical account, see Morantz 1974. For an epidemiological description, see the National Health Survey 1977. Mishler et al. 1981 and Lain Entralgo 1969 provide discussions of the social context within and around the doctor-patient relationship.

2 Suits have been brought against physicians for failure to treat DES-related cancers along with many other kinds of cancer, but these are negligence cases, and the relation of the cancer to the prescription of DES is not an issue. One very early case against a prescribing physician in Pennsylvania was brought in order to obtain release of a patient's records, not for the actual prescription of DES. It is the opinion of legal experts that doctors would not be liable for prescribing DES because it was usual and customary practice to do so. There are now several "grandchild" suits against drug companies on behalf of defective infants born prematurely to mothers with uterine anomalies that contributed to incompetent cervices and early delivery. (Personal communications with lawyers Paul Rheingold of New York and Frederic A. Bremseth of Minneapolis, and with William Keough of *DES Litigation Reporter,* December 1983.)

3 Monologuist Cornelia Otis Skinner (1955) entitled her address to the College of Obstetricians and Gynecologists "Bottoms Up!" In it she describes three types of gynecologist: the silent one, the crooner who sings through the examination, and the chatty one who seems so intimate but never recognizes the patient's face. Her way of preserving dignity when told at the gynecologic examination to "take off everything except shoes and stockings" was to keep her hat on.

4 According to gynecologist John Vallee, an adequate examination can be performed with the patient's legs in stirrups while she sits up (personal communication, November 1983). For historical and sociological accounts of examina-

tion techniques and their consequences for the woman patient, see Emerson 1970; Smith-Rosenberg and Rosenberg 1973; Smith-Rosenberg 1974; Tyrone 1952; and Wood 1973. Comedienne Joan Rivers satirizes the experience of a pelvic examination in a monologue on her record "What Becomes a Semi-Legend Most."

Males examined in the lithotomy position describe strong anxiety feelings.

5 Nadelson et al. (1982) discuss female aggression from a psychoanalytic point of view. Hennig and Jardim (1978) show how inhibition of aggression affects the behavior of women in the business world. Gilligan (1982) postulates that a different developmental path for aggression in females can be adaptive and salutory. For discussions of patient compliance unrelated to gender, see Blackwell 1973 and Davis 1978.

6 For material related to the socialization of women patients, see Bell 1979; Corea 1977; Ehrenreich and English 1973; Hartman and Banner 1974; Moulton 1977; and Ruzek 1978.

Chapter 7

1 See Newton 1973; ACOG Newsletters, May 1973, January 1975, October 1975, April 1977, and November 1978; and ACOG Technical Bulletin, May 1973. *American Family Physician* (1979) asked family doctors to be alert to DES cases, as ACOG had earlier asked obstetrician-gynecologists; the journal called attention to the NCI publications available to physicians.

There is an interesting difference in methods of casefinding between the United States and the United Kingdom, perhaps reflecting a difference in medical philosophy and ethics. The United States approach has been to reach the consumer directly, via doctors and the media, and to obtain medical information from doctors only with the patient's consent. By contrast, the British method has been to inform physicians and to leave it to the discretion of the general practitioners to treat DES-exposed individuals appropriately. Vessey et al. (1983) did their follow-up study in Britain under the direction of a Medical Research Council working group. The group members ruled that the researchers should have no direct contact with the mothers who took DES or their offspring, so as not to arouse anxiety. All their work was therefore done indirectly and without the patients' knowledge. They used medical records, cancer registries, and postal questionnaires to general practitioners whose patient rosters are centrally recorded.

2 Alice Hamm, personal communication, 9 February 1982.

3 Discussions of iatrogenesis can be found in Illich 1975, a polemical commentary on the medical system, and Smithells 1975, a commentary from within the medical community.

4 Discussions of error, uncertainty, and ambiguity in medical training are found in Barrows 1968; Bosk 1979; Bursztajn et al. 1981; Fox 1957; Glauber 1953; Millman 1977; and Werner and Schneider 1974.

5 For material relevant to this topic, see Eichna 1980; Friedson 1972; Knowles 1968; Krakowski 1979; and Newton, Reader, and Kendall 1957.

6 In a personal interview (November 1983), Dr. DeGroot compared casefinding in the thyroid and DES situations. For further technical elaboration see De-Groot and Paloyan 1973. A symposium edited by DeGroot et al. (1977) documents the programs for and problems in casefinding for radiation-induced thyroid cancer.

7 In Frazier 1971, Mrs. Billy Graham is reported to have said: "If I were an actress who was going to play, let's say, Joan of Arc, I would learn all there is to learn about Joan of Arc. And if I were a doctor or anyone else trying to play God, I would learn all I could about God." On the physician as God, see also Augenstein 1969 and Osmond 1980.

8 Like all social systems, medical opinion and practice are influenced by qualities of charismatic and persuasive leadership. Medical professionals get caught up in hero worship as does the general public. Naftulin et al. (1973) coined the term "Dr. Fox Effect" to describe the phenomenon of medical educators being taken in by a seeming colleague. They introduced an actor to a group of professional medical educators as Dr. Myron L. Fox, a distinguished, well-credentialed authority. His lecture was filled with double-talk, contradictions, irrelevancies, and a few good jokes. Nevertheless, ratings of audience satisfaction were quite high.

9 Responses to Relman's editorial, "Here Come the Women" (*New England Journal of Medicine*, 29 May 1980), suggest that the impact of women on medicine and of medicine on women is neither so simple nor so hopeful as he believes (*New England Journal of Medicine*, 11 September 1980; see also Spiro 1975).

10 Classic works on patient care are Putnam 1899; Peabody 1927; and Balint 1964.

11 On Semmelweis, see *Encyclopedia Brittanica*, vol. 20, 1972; and Thompson 1940. For a primary document, see Semmelweis 1861.

12 See Anderson and Turnbull, in Enkin and Chalmers 1982, pp. 163–81, on the effects of estrogens, progestogens, and beta-mimetics in pregnancy. Beta-mimetic drugs have been widely tested with inconsistent results. They relax uterine contractions, delay labor, and thus allow the fetus to develop. Examples of such drugs are ritodrine and terbutaline. Bendectin, a drug used to control nausea and vomiting in pregnancy, has been the focus of recent controversy around birth defects. Other drugs that have been approved in recent years and have aroused serious concern are Oraflex (benoxaprofen), Zomax (zomepirac), and Selacryn (ticrynafen).

13 Dr. Herbert W. Horne, Jr., personal communication, 29 November 1982.

Chapter 8

1 Katz 1972 is the standard textbook on experimentation with human beings. Winston et al. 1982 provide an interesting case example of informed consent. For important debates on medical experimentation, see Katz 1972; Barber et

al. 1973; Eisenberg 1977; Freund 1970; Fried 1974; Guttentag 1953; and Ramsey 1975. Special concerns are raised by research on human beings affecting the fetus; see Ramsey 1975 and Singer 1976. Social responsibility in the field of obstetrics and gynecology is addressed in Barnes 1965. Mishler 1979, Starr 1983, and Conrad and Schneider 1980 discuss the social factors in medical practice. On medical ethics, see the Hastings Center Report (available from the Hastings Center, 360 Broadway, Hastings-on-Hudson, N.Y. 10706); Beecher 1966; Brody 1973; and Perl and Shelp 1982. Medical mistakes are the subject of Bosk 1979 and Paget 1978. Reflective writings on the nature of medicine as science are Bronowski 1959, 1977; Chargaff 1973, 1976; Dubos 1959; and Popper 1962.

2 See, for example, Public Citizen Health Research Group, 2000 P Street N.W., Washington, D.C. 20036.

Glossary

Abortion. Premature stoppage of the pregnancy process. A spontaneous abortion is also called a *miscarriage*. *Habitual abortion* is defined as loss of a nonviable fetus in three or more successive pregnancies. *Threatened abortion* is a condition in which there is bloody discharge from the uterus and the continuity of the pregnancy is in doubt.

Adenocarcinoma. A cancer in which the malignant cells take the form of glands.

Adenosis. Glandular tissue occurring in unexpected places; e.g., glands similar to those normally found on the inside of the uterus occurring on the outside of the cervix and in the vagina.

Adolescence. Technically, the stage of life that starts with the appearance of secondary sex characteristics (e.g., breasts for females, facial hair for males) and ends when the body stops growing.

Adrenocorticotrophic hormone (ACTH). A naturally occurring pituitary hormone that stimulates cortisone production and is used therapeutically to enhance the body's cortisone level.

Amenorrhea. Absence of menses.

Androgen. A substance that produces masculinization, such as the hormone from the male testes.

Anecdotal series. Evidence based on personal impressions rather than measurement.

Anomalies. Deviations from the norm, as in the structure of a part of the body—for example, the cervix.

Anorexia. Loss or decrease in appetite. *Anorexia nervosa* is a condition that affects young women in particular and is characterized by progressive and often extreme weight loss, obsessions with food, and emotional problems.

Beta-mimetic drugs. Drugs that mimic certain actions of the sympathetic nervous system; e.g., that raise blood pressure, increase heart rate, increase blood sugar, and inhibit contractions of the uterus.

Biopsy. Removal and microscopic examination of tissue from a live patient for the purpose of diagnosis.

Bleeding. Letting of blood for therapeutic purposes.

Blind study. A research evaluation in which neither the investigator nor the patient knows which treatment is being given at the time it is given.

Carcinogen. A cancer-producing substance.

Carcinoma. Malignant growth composed of epithelial cells that spreads to other tissues. *Carcinoma in situ* refers to early malignant growth that is still in place and has not spread to surrounding tissues.

Cautery. The process of killing tissue by heat produced by either electricity or a caustic substance.

Cervix. The narrow lower end of the uterus that can be seen and felt in the vagina.

Chemotherapy. Chemical treatment of disease (e.g., cancer) designed to affect diseased sites with minimal injury to the rest of the person.

Chromosome. The entity within the cell nucleus that contains hereditary factors (genes).

Clitoridectomy. Removal of the clitoris, the small erectile body at the front of the female genitals that is the female homolog of the penis.

Colposcopy. Procedure for examination of the vagina and cervix with a viewer (colposcope) which magnifies these organs to the examiner's eye.

Columnar cells. Tall cells shaped like columns, normally lining the uterine cavity.

Congenital. Existing at or before birth.

Conization. The removal of a cone of tissue from the cervix, a surgical therapy for *carcinoma in situ.*

Control group. A group similar to a test population in all conditions except the one factor being studied.

Cortisone. A hormone naturally produced by the cortex of the adrenal gland. It is used in natural and synthetic forms (also called *steroids*) to treat numerous diseases, such as those characterized by inflammation.

Diabetes. A disorder in which the person cannot metabolize carbohydrates because of a deficiency in insulin production from the pancreas.

Dialysis. A process that separates solids in solution by their slower rate of passing through a semipermeable membrane. *Renal dialysis* is a procedure that filters toxins from the blood in people whose kidneys cannot adequately do so.

Dysplasia. Development of abnormal tissue.

Dysmenorrhea. Painful or difficult menses.

Eclampsia. Convulsions and/or coma in a pregnant woman or one who has just delivered, associated with high blood pressure, swelling, and protein in the urine.

Ectopic pregnancy. Pregnancy that occurs in an abnormal place in the uterus, usually in the fallopian tube instead of in the body of the uterus. Such a pregnancy must be terminated prematurely to keep the tube from rupturing.

Ectropion. An abnormality of the cervix in which the edge turns outward. Synonymous with *eversion*.

Edema. An excessive accumulation of fluid in cells, tissues, and body cavities; from Greek *oidema,* meaning a swelling.

Electron microscopy. Use of a high-magnification (around a million times) microscope that produces magnified images with electrons rather than visible light, making it possible to view objects smaller than the wavelength of light.

Embryo. An organism in the early stage of development; in the human, from one week after conception to the end of the second month.

Endocrinology. The scientific study of the internal secretions or hormones.

Endometrium. The mucous membrane lining the uterus.

Epidemiology. Study of the factors and determinants governing the frequency and distribution of disease.

Epithelium. The type of tissue that covers the internal and external surfaces of the body, including such small cavities as the mouth and vagina.

Estrogen. A generic term for naturally occurring and synthetic substances that promote *estrus* and stimulate the development of secondary sex characteristics in the female.

Estrus. An intermittent period of intense sexual excitement in female mammals, excluding humans, during which conception can occur.

Ethical drugs. A term used by drug manufacturers to distinguish prescription drugs from patent, or proprietary, medicines, which can be sold over the counter.

Eversion. See *Ectropion.*

Excision. Removal of a pathological area by cutting it out.

Fetus. The developing human within the mother's uterus, between two months (end of the embryonic period) and birth.

Gonad. A gland that produces seed for procreation, the ovary in the female and the testis in the male.

Gonorrhea. A contagious inflammation of mucous membranes transmitted chiefly by sex (i.e., a venereal disease), caused by a bacterium. In the female it may be present without producing symptoms and thus can be unwittingly transmitted to her sexual partner or infant.

Gynecology. The branch of medicine that studies diseases and hygiene of the genital tract in women.

Hemangioma. A benign tumor, such as a strawberry birthmark, made up of newly formed blood vessels.

Hemophilia. A hereditary blood clotting disorder causing problems of hemorrhage, usually found in males and inherited through the mother.

Histochemistry. Study of the chemical composition and reactivity of body tissues.

Hormone. A natural chemical substance secreted by an endocrine gland (or a synthetic one that resembles it) that circulates in the body fluids and specifically stimulates other organs.

Hot flashes. The expression coined by the medical profession to describe the experier e of heat and flushing of women going through menopause.

Human menopausal gonadotrophins (HMG). Pituitary hormones sometimes used as a medic on to induce ovulation.

Hypophysis. The pituitary gland, which regulates secretion of hormones from sex glands and other endocrine organs.

Hysterectomy. Surgical removal of the uterus.

Hysterosalpingogram. X-ray study of the uterus and fallopian tubes after the injection of opaque material that makes visible the contour of the inner cavity.

Immunochemistry. The scientific study of the chemical reactions of the body's immune system, which protects against infection.

Intrauterine device (IUD). A type of female contraceptive that is inserted into the uterine cavity through the cervical opening.

In utero. Literally, within the uterus; pertaining to the time of embryonic and fetal growth.

Lactation. The secretion of milk.

Laparoscopy. The insertion of the equivalent of a telescope with a light source into the abdomen in order to look around at various organs.

Laser treatment. A procedure using a laser (*l*ight *a*mplification by *s*imulated *e*mission of *r*adiation), a device that creates highly amplified coherent visible light that can be directed at specific body areas to destroy abnormal tissue.

Lithotomy. The position used for pelvic examination in the United States: the woman places her legs in stirrups, spread apart, while she lies on her back on the examining table. The term originally meant the removal of a stone by cutting into the bladder.

Mastoid. The nipple-shaped bone behind the ear.

Megalomania. The irrational conviction of one's greatness, goodness, or power.

Menarche. The beginning of menstrual function, which takes place around puberty.

Menopause. The naturally occurring cessation of menstruation in human females, generally between the ages of forty-five and fifty-four.

Mesonephric ducts. The embryonic excretory organ, first described by Kaspar Friedrich Wolff (1733–94); also termed *wolffian cells.*

Metaplasia. The transformation of fully differentiated tissue of one kind into fully differentiated tissue of another kind.

Miscarriage. See *Abortion.*

Müllerian ducts and tubercle. Embryonic structures that are precursors of the urogenital tract; named by Johannes Peter Müller, distinguished German physiologist (1801–58).

Neonatal asphyxia. Suffocation of an infant within the first month of life. Asphyxia (literally, "without pulse") can occur when the placenta separates prematurely and does not provide adequate oxygen to the baby. A *neonate* (newborn) can have compromised oxygen flow to the vital organs for many reasons; e.g., mechanical problems in labor and delivery, immaturity of the breathing system.

Neonatologist. A pediatrician trained in the disorders and care of the newborn.

Neoplasia. The formation of any new and abnormal growth, such as a tumor.

Obstetrics. The branch of surgery that deals with the management of pregnancy, labor, delivery, and the period immediately following.

Oncology. A subspecialty of internal medicine that involves the study of tumors.

Ovaries. In the human female, the two flat, oval-shaped sexual glands to each side of the uterus in which eggs (*ova*) are formed.

Ovulation. The periodic release of a mature ovum from the ovary.

Osteoporosis. Abnormal porousness and thinning of bone, commonly affecting post-menopausal women.

Pap smear. A test named for Dr. George Papanicolau that has become part of a routine gynecological examination. Scrapings of the superficial cervical and vaginal cells are examined microscopically for changes that can suggest early cancer. The procedure has become a major technique for spotting cancerous and precancerous cervical conditions.

Patent drug. See *Proprietary drug.*

Placebo. An inactive substance originally given for the purpose of "pleasing the patient" by making him believe he was being treated, now used in medical research to measure the effect of a more specific medication or treatment by comparison.

Placebo effect. Genuine beneficial effect from *placebo.* The term came into use during the Allied landing in Italy in World War II, when a shortage of morphine existed and soldiers with real injuries and real pain experienced relief from injections of inactive, nonpharmacologic liquids (Dr. Samuel Shapiro, personal communication, 14 March 1984).

Placenta. The vascular organ that develops within the uterus in pregnancy and acts as a network of communication between the mother and the fetus, via the umbilical cord.

Progesterone. A hormone produced by the *corpus luteum,* a mass of endocrine tissue in the ovary, that prepares the uterine lining for implantation of a fertilized ovum.

Prophylaxis. The prevention of disease.

Proprietary drug. According to the American Medical Association, a nonprescription, over-the-counter medication used in the treatment of disease and "protected against free competition as to name, product, composition, or process of manufacture by secrecy, patent, trade mark or copyright, or by any other means." Also called a *patent drug.*

Prostate. A gland in the male that surrounds the urethra and neck of the bladder. A prevalent site of cancer that has responded to estrogen or antiandrogen treatment.

Puberty. The period of human development when reproductive organs begin to function, making reproduction possible.

Randomized clinical trial (RCT). A method of testing a new drug or procedure in which the treatment is given to a group of people chosen at random (with minimal bias) and its effects are compared to the effects of no treatment or an established treatment administered to a comparable randomly selected group.

Regression. The usually temporary return to an earlier state of development.

Retrolental fibroplasia (RLF). Abnormal growth of tissue behind the lens of the eyes in newborns that often progresses to blindness.

Squamous cells. Flat cells found on the skin surfaces of the body and lining all mucous membranes of body orifices.

Squamous dysplasia. Abnormal development of *squamous cells,* which may be discovered, for example, during a routine Pap smear showing suspicious changes on the top layer of the epithelium of the mucous membrane.

Squamous metaplasia. The change that adenosis tissue usually undergoes after puberty to become normal squamous epithelium.

Steroid. One of several compounds resembling cholesterol, including the natural sex hormones (*estrogen, progesterone, testosterone*), bile acids, and some carcinogenic hydrocarbons.

Stillbirth. The birth of a dead child after twenty weeks' gestation.

Subfertility. Less than average ability to conceive and bear a child.

Sulfa. A drug used to treat infection before penicillin and antibiotics came into widespread use after World War II. Many sulfa-type drugs are still in use—e.g., for urinary tract infections.

Teratogenic. Something that produces physical abnormalities and defects during the development of the embryo and fetus. Literally, "monster-making."

Thalidomide. A drug used in Europe around 1960 for treatment of nausea, vomiting, and insomnia in pregnancy; it produced severe congenital limb deformities in the developing child and was never approved for use in the United States.

Thymus. A glandlike body related to immunity and situated high in the chest near the neck; it is of maximum size in early childhood and tends to disappear or become rudimentary with maturity.

Toxemia. A metabolic disturbance of pregnancy characterized by *edema* and an increase in blood pressure; the condition can proceed to *eclampsia*.

Transference. The shifting of feelings related to previously important figures in one's life onto a currently important person, such as a doctor.

Trauma. Unexpected and undesired experience that disrupts the sense of bodily and/or psychological integrity.

Tubal pregnancy. See *Ectopic pregnancy*.

Urethra. The tube through which urine travels from the bladder to the outside of the body. In the male seminal ejaculations are also conveyed by the urethra.

Urogenital sinus. The area in the embryo from which the urinary and genital apparatus derives.

Uterus. In the human female, a hollow, muscular pear-shaped organ approximately three inches long consisting of a broad, flat part (body) above, tapering to a narrow, cylindrical part (cervix) below. Between *menarche* and *menopause* a lining (*endometrium*) develops and is shed each month in *menstruation*. The uterus is the home that nourishes the developing embryo and fetus in pregnancy.

Vagina. A sheathlike structure in the female extending from the cervix to the labia. It receives the penis in sexual intercourse and is the birth canal for the baby's passage from the uterus to the outside world.

Vaginectomy. Surgical removal of the vagina.

Vaginitis. Inflammation and irritation of the vagina, characterized by itching, pain, and discharge, usually caused by an infectious agent. *Senile* or *atrophic vaginitis* is irritation caused after menopause by decreased production of estrogen and vaginal use.

Weeding. Removal by excision of scattered areas of adenosis—as in weeding a garden.

Wolffian cells. See *Mesonephric ducts*.

Bibliography

Aberle, S., and Corner, W. 1953. *Twenty-five years of sex research: History of the National Research Council Committee for Research into Problems of Sex, 1922–1947*. Philadelphia: Saunders.

Allen, E., Danforth, H., and Doisy, A., eds. 1939. *Sex and internal secretions: A survey of recent research*, 2d ed. Baltimore: Williams and Wilkins.

American College of Obstetricians and Gynecologists. Newsletters of May 1973, January 1975, October 1975, April 1977, and November 1978. Items on DES. Suite 300 East, 600 Maryland Ave. SW., Washington, D.C. 20024–2588.

――――. 1973. *Maternal stilbestrol-genital adenocarcinoma and follow-up of exposed young women*. Technical Bulletin no. 22, May.

American Family Physician. 1977. NCI Pamphlet discusses effects of DES exposure in utero. *Am. Fam. Phys. News* 16: 271–72.

Anderson, B., Watring, W. G., Edinger, Jr., D. D., Small, E. C., Neiland, A. T., and Safah, H. 1979. Development of DES-associated clear-cell carcinoma: The importance of regular screening. *Ob. Gyn.* 53: 293–99.

Antonioli, D. A., Burke, L., and Friedman, E. A. 1980. Natural history of diethystilbestrol-associated genital tract lesions: Cervical ectopy and cervicovaginal hood. *Am. J. Ob. Gyn.* 137: 847–53.

Apfel, R. J. 1982. How are women sicker than men? An overview of psychosomatic problems in women. *Psychother. Psychosom.* 37: 106–18.

Aristotle. 1941. *Basic Works of Aristotle*, ed. Richard McKeon. New York: Random House.

Aschheim, S. 1935. Pregnancy tests. *JAMA* 104: 1324–1329.

Augenstein, L. G. 1969. *Come, let us play god*. New York: Harper and Row.

Aycock, W. L. 1942. Tonsillectomy and poliomyelitis. *Medicine* 21:65–94.

Baker, S. W., and Ehrhardt, A. 1974. Prenatal androgen, intelligence, and cognitive sex differences. In *Sex differences in behavior*, ed. R. C. Friedman. New York: John Wiley.

Balint, M. 1964. *The doctor, his patient and the illness*. 2d ed. New York: International Universities Press.

Banbury Report no. 8. 1981. *Hormones & Breast Cancer*, ed. Pike, M. C., Siiteri, P. K., and Welsch, C. W. New York: Cold Spring Harbor Laboratory.

Banta, H. D., and Behney, C. J. 1981. Policy formulation and technology assessment. *Milbank Mem. Fund Q.: Health and Society* 59: 445–79.

Banta, H. D., and Thacker, S. B. 1979. Policies toward medical technology: The case of electronic fetal monitoring. *Am. J. P. H.* 69: 931–35.

Barber, B., Lally, J. J., Makarushka, J. L., and Sullivan, D. 1973. *Research on human subjects: Problems of social control in medical experimentation*. New York: Russell Sage.

Barnes, A. B. 1979. Menstrual history of young women exposed *in utero* to diethystilbestrol. *Fertility and Sterility* 32: 148–53.

Barnes, A. B., Colton, T., Gundersen, J., Noller, K. L., Tilley, B. C., Strama, T., Townsend, D. E., Hatab, P., and O'Brien, P. 1980. Fertility and outcome of pregnancy in women exposed *in utero* to diethylstilbestrol. *New Eng. J. Med.* 302: 609–13.

Barnes, A. C., ed. 1965. *The social responsibility of gynecology and obstetrics*. Baltimore: John Hopkins University Press.

Barnes, R. 1890. On the correlations of sexual functions and mental disorders of women. *Brit. Gyn. J.* 6: 390–430.

Barrows, H. S. 1968. Simulated patients in medical teaching. *Can. Med. Assn. J.* 98: 674–76.

Bassuk, E. L. 1983. "Normal" ovariotomy, 1872–1893: Sadism or humanitarian health care. Unpublished manuscript presented at Bunting Institute, Radcliffe College, 8 March 1983, Cambridge, Mass.

Becker, H. S., Gerr, B., Hughes, E. C., and Strauss, A. L. 1961. *Boys in white: Student culture in medical school*. Chicago: University of Chicago Press.

Beecher, H. K. 1966. Ethics and clinical research. *New Eng. J. Med.* 274: 1354–1360.

Bell, S. E. 1979. Political gynecology: Gynecological imperialism and the politics of self-help. *Science for the People,* September–October: 8–14.

———. 1980. The synthetic compound diethylstilbestrol (DES) 1938–1941: The social construction of a medical treatment. Ph.D. dissertation, Brandeis University.

———. 1984. A new model of medical technology development: A case study of DES. In *Research in the sociology of health care,* ed. J. Roth and S. Ruzek, vol. 4. Greenwich, Ct.: JAI Press.

Belsky, D. E. 1978. DES daughters: Adaptation to bodily uncertainty. Unpublished manuscript based on independent investigation for degree of Master of Social Work, Smith College School for Social Work.

Beral, V., and Colwell, L. 1980. Randomized trial of high doses of stilboestrol and ethisterone in pregnancy: Long-term follow-up of mothers. *Brit. Med. J.* 281: 1098–1101.

Beral, V., and Colwell, L. 1981. Randomized trial of high doses of stilboestrol & ethisterone therapy in pregnancy: Long-term follow-up of the children. *J. Epid. Com. Health.* 35: 155–60.

Berger, M. J., and Goldstein, D. P. 1980. Impaired reproductive performance in DES-exposed women. *Ob. Gyn.* 55: 25–27.

Bertin, C. 1982. *Marie Bonaparte: A life.* New York: Harcourt Brace Jovanovich.

Bibbo, M., Ali, I., Al-Naqeeb, M., Baccarini, I., Climaco, L. A., Gill, W., Sonek, M., and Wied, G. L. 1975. Cytologic findings in female and male offspring of DES-treated mothers. *Acta Cytol.* 19: 568–72.

Bibbo, M., Al-Naqeeb, M., Baccarini, I., Gill, W., Newton, M., Sleeper, K. M., Sonek, M., and Wied, G. L. 1975. Follow-up study of male and female offspring of DES-treated mothers: A preliminary report. *J. Reprod. Med.* 15: 29–32.

Bibbo, M., Gill, W. B., Azizi, F., Blough, R., Fang, V. S., Rosenfeld, R. L., Schumacher, G. F. B., Sleeper, K., Sonek, M. G., and Wied, G. L. 1977. Follow-up study of male and female offspring of DES-exposed mothers. *Ob. Gyn.* 49: 1–8.

Bibbo, M., Haenszel, W. M., Wied, G. L., Hubby, M., and Herbst, A. L. 1978. A twenty-five year follow-up study of women exposed to diethylstilbestrol during pregnancy. *New Eng. J. Med.* 298: 763–67.

Bibring, G., Dwyer, T., Huntington, D., and Valenstein, A. F. 1961. A study of the earliest mother-child relationship. *Psychoanal. Stud. Child.* 16: 9–72.

Bichler, J. 1981. *DES daughter: The Joyce Bichler story.* New York: Avon.

Bishop, P. M. F., Boycott, M., and Zuckerman, S. 1939. The oestrogenic properties of "stilboestrol" (diethylstilboestrol). *Lancet* 1: 5–11.

Blackwell, B. 1973. Drug therapy: Patient compliance. *New Eng. J. Med.* 289: 249–52.

Blaikey, J. B., Dewhurst, C. J., Ferreira, H. P., and Lewis, T. L. T. 1971. Vaginal adenosis: Clinical and pathological features with special references to malignant change. *J. Ob. Gyn. Br. Commonw.* 78: 1115–1122.

Blair, P. B. 1981. Immunologic considerations of early exposure of experimental rodents to diethylstilbestrol and steroid hormones. In Herbst and Bern 1981, pp. 167–78.

Bologh, R. W. 1981. Grounding the alienation of self and body: A critical, phenomenological analysis of the patient in western medicine. *Sociology of Health and Illness* 3: 188–206.

Bongiovanni, A. M., DiGeorge, A. M., and Grumback, M. M. 1959. Masculinization of the female infant associated with estrogenic therapy alone during gestation: Four cases. *J. Clin. Endocr.* 19: 1004–1010.

Bosk, C. L. 1979. *Forgive and remember: Managing medical failure.* Chicago: University of Chicago Press.

Brackbill, Y., and Berendes, H. W. 1978. Dangers of diethylstilboestrol: Review of a 1953 paper. *Lancet* 2: 520.

Brian, D. D., Tilley, B. C., Labarthé, D. R., O'Fallon, W. M., Noller, K. L., and Kurland, L. T. 1980. Breast cancer in DES-exposed mothers: Absence of association. *Mayo Clin. Proc.* 55: 89–93.

Brody, H. 1973. The systems view of man: Implications for medicine, science, and ethics. *Perspect. Biol. Med.* 17: 71–92.

Bronowski, J. 1959. *The common sense of science.* New York: Random House.

–––––. 1977. *A sense of the future.* Cambridge: MIT Press.

Burdick, H. O., and Vedder, H. 1941. The effect of stilbestrol in early pregnancy. *Endocrinology* 28: 629–32.

Burgess, A. W., and Holmstrom, L. L. 1974. Rape trauma syndrome. *Am. J. Psychiatry* 131: 981–86.

Burghardt, E., and Holzer, E. 1980. Treatment of carcinoma in situ: Evaluation of 1609 cases. *Ob. Gyn.* 55: 539–45.

Burke, L., Antonioli, D., and Friedman, E. A. 1981. Evolution of diethylstilbestrol-associated genital tract lesions. *Ob. Gyn.* 57: 79–84.

Burke, L., Antonioli, D., Knapp, R. C., and Friedman, E. A. 1974. Vaginal adenosis: Correlation of colposcopic and pathologic findings. *Ob. Gyn.* 44: 257–64.

Burke, L., Apfel, R. J., Fisher, S. M., and Shaw, J. G. 1980. Observations on the psychological impact of diethylstilbestrol exposure and suggestions on management. *J. Reprod. Med.* 24: 99–102.

Burnham, J. 1982. American medicine's golden age: What happened to it? *Science* 215: 1474–1479.

Burroughs, W. 1956. Method of raising beef cattle and sheep and feed rations for use therein. Application to the U.S. Patent Office for use of DES as growth stimulant in cattle feed. Patented 19 June 1956.

Burroughs, W., Culbertson, C. C., Kastelic, J., Cheng, E., and Hale, W. H. 1954. The effects of trace amounts of diethylstilbestrol in rations of fattening steers. *Science* 120: 266–67.

Bursztajn, H., Hamm, R. M., Feinbloom, R. I., and Brodsky, A. 1981. *Medical choices, medical chances: How patients' families and physicians can cope with uncertainty.* New York: Delacorte.

Butendant, A. 1929. Untersuchungen über das weibliche Sexualhormon: Darstellung und Eigenschaften des Kristallisierten "Progynons." *Deutsche Med. Wchnschr.* 55: 2171ff.

Buxton, C. L., and Engle, E. T. 1939. Effects of the therapeutic use of diethylstilbestrol. *JAMA* 113: 2318–2320.

Byar, D. P., Simon, R. M., Friedewald, W. T., Schiesselman, J. J., Demets, D. L., Ellenberg, J. H., Gail, M. H., and Ware, J. H. 1976. Randomized clinical trials: Perspectives on some recent ideas. *New Eng. J. Med.* 295: 74–80.

Byrne, P. S., and Long, B. E. L. 1976. *Doctors talking to patients.* London: HMSO.

Califano, Jr., J. A. 1978. Statement of October 4 by Secretary of Health, Education and Welfare in HEW news regarding Task Force Report.

Canario, E. M., Houston, G., and Smith, C. A. 1953. Postnatal growth and development of infants born after diethylstilbestrol administration during pregnancy. *Am. J. Ob. Gyn.* 65: 1298–1304.

Chalmers, I. 1976. British debate on obstetric practice. *Pediatrics* 58: 308–12.

——. 1983. Scientific inquiry and authoritarianism in perinatal care and education. *Birth* 10: 151–66.

Chalmers, T. C. 1974. The impact of controlled trials on the practice of medicine. *Mt. Sinai J. Med.* 41: 753–58.

——. 1975. Randomization: Perils and problems (letter). *New Eng. J. Med.* 292: 1036–1037.

Chalmers, T. C., Celano, P., Sacks, H. S., and Smith, Jr., H. 1983. Bias in treatment assignment in controlled clinical trials. *New Eng. J. Med.* 309: 1358–1361.

Chargaff, E. 1973. Bitter fruits from the tree of knowledge: Remarks on the current revulsion from science. *Persp. Biol. Med.* 16: 486–502.

Chargaff, E. 1976. Triviality in science: A brief meditation on fashions. *Persp. Biol. Med.* 19: 324–33.

———. 1982. Hysteria and women. *Amer. J. Psychiatry* 139: 545–51.

Chodorow, N. 1978. *The reproduction of mothering*. Berkeley and Los Angeles: University of California Press.

Clark, A. C. 1888. Relations of the sexual and reproductive functions to insanity. *Am. J. Insanity* 45: 292–97.

Clifford, S. H. 1964. High risk pregnancy: Prevention of prematurity, the *sine qua non* for reduction of mental retardation and other neurologic disorders. *New Eng. J. Med.* 271: 243–49.

Cohler, B. J., and Grunebaum, H. U. 1981. *Mothers, grandmothers and daughters*. New York: Wiley.

Coleman, J., Katz, E., Menzel, H. 1957. The diffusion of innovation among physicians. *Sociometry.* 20: 253–70.

Colvin, E. D., Bartholomew, R. A., Grimes, W. H., and Fish, J. 1950. Salvage possibilities in threatened abortion. *Am. J. Ob. Gyn.* 59: 1208–1224.

Conley, G. R., Sant, G. R., Ucci, A. A., and Mitcheson, H. D. 1983. Seminoma and epididymal cysts in a young man with known diethylstilbestrol exposure in utero. *JAMA* 249: 1325–1326.

Conrad, P., and Schneider, J. W. 1980. Looking at levels of medicalization: A comment on Strong's critique of the thesis of medical imperialism. *Social Science and Medicine* 14A: 75–79.

Consumer Reports. September 1980. Carcinogen used in cattle despite federal ban. P. 529.

Cook, S. 1981. *Second life*. New York: Simon and Schuster.

Copelson, M., Pixley, E., and Reid, B. 1971. *Colposcopy*. Springfield, Il.: Charles C. Thomas.

Corea, G. 1977. *The hidden malpractice: How American medicine treats women as patients and professionals*. New York: William Morrow.

Cosgrove, M. D., Benton, B., and Henderson, B. E. 1977. Male genitourinary abnormalities and maternal diethylstilbestrol. *J. Urology* 117: 220–22.

Cousins, L., Karp, W., Lacey, C., and Lucas, W. E. 1980. Reproductive outcomes of women exposed to diethylstilbestrol in utero. *Ob. Gyn.* 56: 70–76.

Cousins, N., ed. 1982. *The physician in literature.* Philadelphia: Saunders.

Crowder, R. E., Bills, E. S., and Broadbent, J. S. 1950. The management of threatened abortion: A study of 100 cases. *Am. J. Ob. Gyn.* 60: 896–99.

Cunha, G. R. 1976. Epithelial-stromal interactions in development of the urogenital tract. *Int. Rev. Cytol.* 47: 137–94.

Davis, M. 1978. Variations in patients' compliance with doctors' advice: An empirical analysis of patterns of communication. *Am. J. Pub. Health* 58: (2): 274–88.

Davis, M. E. 1940. A clinical study of stilbestrol. *Am. J. Ob. Gyn.* 39: 1938–1953.

Davis, M. E., and Fugo, N. W. 1950. Steroids in the treatment of early pregnancy complications. *JAMA* 142: 778–85.

DeCherney, A. H., and Berkowitz, G. S. 1982. Female fecundity and age. *New Eng. J. Med.* 306: 424–26.

DeCherney, A. H., Cholst, I., Naftolin, F. 1981. Structure and function of the Fallopian tube following exposure to diethylstilbestrol (DES) during gestation. *Fertil. Steril.* 36: 741–45.

Deckert, G. H. 1976. Keynote speech at annual meetings of the Association for Academic Psychiatry, February.

DeGroot, L. J., Frohman, L. A., Kaplan, E. L., and Refetoff, S., 1977, eds. *Radiation-associated thyroid carcinoma.* New York: Grune and Stratton.

DeGroot, L. J., and Paloyan, E. 1973. Thyroid carcinoma and radiation: A Chicago endemic. *JAMA* 225: 487–91.

Dennerstein, L., and Burrows, G. D. 1983. *Handbook of psychosomatic obstetrics and gynecology.* Amsterdam: Elsevier.

DerSimonian, R., Charette, L. J., McPeek, B., and Mosteller, F. 1982. Reporting on methods in clinical trials. *New Eng. J. Med.* 306: 1332–1337.

DES Action Voice. Quarterly publication of DES Action National, Inc. East Coast office: Long Island Jewish–Hillside Medical Center, New Hyde Park, N.Y. 11040; West Coast office: 1638-B Haight St., San Francisco, Ca. 94117.

DES Litigation Reporter. Andrews Publishing Co., P. O. Box 200, Edgemont, Pa. 19028. Tel. (215) 353-2565.

DES National Quarterly. Published by DES Registry, Inc., 5426 27th St. NW, Washington, D.C. 20015.

DES Task Force. 1978. Summary report, 21 September. NIH pub. no. 82–1688. Reprinted October 1981. Available from U.S. Department of Health and Human Services, National Institutes of Health, Rockville, Md. 20014.

Dieckmann, W. J. 1952. *The toxemias of pregnancy.* 2d ed. St. Louis: C. V. Mosby.

Dieckmann, W. J., Davies, M. E., Rynkiewicz, L. M., and Pottinger, R. E. 1953. Does the administration of diethylstilbestrol during pregnancy have therapeutic value? *Am. J. Ob. Gyn.* 66: 1062–1081.

DiSaia, P. J. 1981. The cervix. In Romney *et al., Gynecology and obstetrics,* New York: McGraw-Hill, pp. 1015–1052.

Dodds, Sir Charles. 1965. *Stilboestrol and after.* In *The scientific basis of medicine,* British Post-Graduate Medical Federation, Annual Reviews. London: Athlone Press.

Dodds, E. C. 1932. The bearing of recent research on the sex hormones on clinical obstetrics and gynecology. *Proc. Royal Soc. Med.* 25: 563–70.

––––––. 1934. The practical outcome of recent research on hormones. *Lancet* 2: 1318–1320.

––––––. 1941. The new oestrogens. *Edinburgh Med. J.* 48: 1–13.

––––––. 1955. Synthetic oestrogens. *Brit. Med. Bull.* 11: 131–34.

Dodds, E. C., Goldberg, L., Lawson, W., and Robinson, R. 1938. Oestrogenic activity of certain synthetic compounds (letter to editor). *Nature* 141: 247–48.

Doisy, E. A. 1941. Glandular physiology and therapy. *JAMA* 116: 501–05.

Doisy, E. A., Veler, E. D., and Thayer, S. 1929. Folliculin from the urine of pregnant women. *Am. J. Physiology* 90: 329–30.

Driscoll, S. G., and Taylor, S. H. 1980. Effects of prenatal maternal estrogen on the male urogenital system. *Ob. Gyn.* 56: 47–50.

Droegemuller, W., Makowski, E. L., and Taylor, E. S. 1970. Vaginal mesonephric adenocarcinoma in two prepubertal children. *Am. J. Dis. Child* 119: 168–70.

Dubos, R. J. 1959. Medical utopias. *Daedalus* 88: 410–24.

Duff, R. S., and Hollingshead, A. B. 1968. *Sickness and society.* New York: Harper and Row.

Dunbar, J. and Stunkard, A. 1979. Adherence to diet and drug regimen. In *Nutrition, lipids and coronary heart disease,* ed. R. Levy et al. New York: Raven Press.

Eaton, W. W., Sigal, J. J., and Weinfeld, M. 1982. Impairment in holocaust survivors after 33 years: Data from an unbiased community sample. *Am. J. Psychiatry* 139: 773–77.

Edward, C. C. 1971. Certain estrogens for oral or parenteral use. *Federal Register* 36: 21537–21538.

Ehrenreich, B., and Ehrenreich, J. 1971. *The American health empire: Power, profits and politics.* New York: Vintage.

Ehrenreich, B., and English, D. 1973. *Complaints and disorders: the sexual politics of sickness.* New York: Feminist Press.

Ehrensaft, D. 1980. When women and men mother. *Socialist Review* 10: 37–74.

Ehrhardt, A. A., and Meyer-Bahlburg, H. F. L. 1981. Effects of prenatal sex hormones on gender-related behavior. *Science* 211: 1312–1318.

Eichna, L. W. 1980. Medical school education, 1975–1979: A student's perspective. *New Eng. J. Med.* 303: 727–34.

Eisenberg, L. 1977. The social imperatives of medical research. *Science* 198: 1105–1110.

Eitinger, L., and Strom, A. 1973. *Mortality and morbidity after excessive stress: A follow-up investigation of Norwegian concentration camp survivors.* New York: Humanities Press.

Elliott, J. 1979. Risk of cancer, dysplasia for DES daughters found "very low." *JAMA* 241: 1555.

Emerson, J. P. 1970. Chapter 3. Behavior in private places: Sustaining definition of reality in gynecological examination. In H. P. Dreitzel, ed., *Recent sociology No. 2: Patterns of communicative behavior,* pp. 74–97. New York: Macmillan.

Engle, E. T., and Crafts, R. C. 1939. Uterine effects from single treatments of stilboestrol and ethinylestradiol in monkeys. *Proc. Soc. Exp. Biol. Med.* 42: 293–96.

Englemann, G. J. 1893. The far-reaching influence of abnormalities of the clitoris. *JAMA* 20: 645.

Enkin, M., and Chalmers, I., eds. 1982. *Effectiveness and satisfaction in antenatal care.* Philadelphia: Lippincott.

Erikson, K. T. 1976. Loss of communality at Buffalo Creek. *Am. J. Psychiatry* 113: 302–05.

FDA drug bulletin. 1971. Quoted in Edward 1971.

FDA drug bulletin. 1978. DES and breast cancer. March–April, p. 10.

Fenichell, S., and Charfoos, L. S. 1982. *Daughters at risk.* New York: Doubleday.

Ferguson, J. H. 1953. Effects of stilbestrol on pregnancy compared to the effect of a placebo. *Am. J. Ob. Gyn.* 65: 592–601.

Fetherston, W. C. 1975. Squamous neoplasia of vagina related to DES syndrome. *Am. J. Ob. Gyn.* 122: 176–81.

Figley, C. R., ed. 1978. *Stress disorders among Vietnam veterans: Theory, research and treatment.* New York: Brunner/Mazel.

Fisher, S. 1967. Motivation for patient delay. *Arch. Gen. Psychiatry.* 16: 676–78.

Fisher, S., and Todd, A., eds. 1982. *The social organization of doctor-patient communication.* Washington, D.C.: Center for Applied Linguistics.

Folkman, J. 1971. Transplacental carcinogenesis by stilbestrol. *New Eng. J. Med.* 285: 404–05.

Forsberg, J. 1972. Estrogen, vaginal cancer and vaginal development. *Am. J. Ob. Gyn.* 113: 83–87.

———. 1976. Animal model of human disease: Adenosis and clear-cell carcinomas of vagina and cervix. *Am. J. Pathology* 84: 669–72.

Fortney, J. A., and Whitehorne, E. W. 1982. The development of an index of high-risk pregnancy. *Am. J. Ob. Gyn.* 143: 501–08.

Fowler, W. C., and Edelman, D. A. 1978. In utero exposure to DES: Evaluation and follow-up of 199 women. *Ob. Gyn.* 51: 459–63.

Fox, R. 1957. Training for uncertainty. Pp. 207–241 in R. K. Newton *et al.* 1957.

Francis, Jr., T., Krill, C. E., Toomey, J. A., and Mack, W. N. 1942. Tonsillectomy in five members of a family. *JAMA* 119: 1392–1396.

Francis, V., Korsch, B. M., Morris, M. J. 1969. Gaps in doctor-patient communication: Patients' response to medical advice. *New Eng. J. Med.* 280: 535–40.

Frankel, R. M. 1980. Talking in interviews: A dispreference for patient-initiated questions in physician-patient encounters. In G. Psathas, J. Coulter, and R. M. Frankel, eds., *Interactional competence,* Norwood, N.J.: Ablex Publishers.

Frazier, C. A., ed. 1971. *Should doctors play God?* Nashville: Broadman Press.

Freidson, E. 1972. *Profession of medicine.* New York: Dodd, Mead.

Freud, A. 1964. The doctor-patient relationship. In Katz 1972.

Freud, A., and Burlingham, D. T. 1944. *Infants without families.* New York: International Universities Press.

Freud, S. 1961. *The standard edition of the complete psychological works of Sigmund Freud,* trans. James Strachey. London: Hogarth.

1911. Psychoanalytic notes on an autobiographical account of a case of paranoia (dementia paranoides). *SE* 12: 3–82.

1923. The ego and the id., chap. 3. *SE* 19: 28–39.

1924. The dissolution of the oedipus complex. *SE* 19: 171–79.

1925. Some psychical consequences of the anatomical distinction between the sexes. *SE* 19: 248–58.

1931. Female sexuality. *SE* 21: 225–43.

Freund, P. A., ed. 1970. *Experimentation with human subjects.* New York: George Braziller, Daedalus Library.

Fried, C. 1974. *Medical experimentation: Personal integrity and social policy.* New York: American Elsevier.

Friedl, E. 1975. *Women and men: An anthropologist's view.* New York: Holt, Rinehart and Winston.

Friday, N. 1977. *My mother myself: The daughter's search for identity.* New York: Dell.

Friedman, M. J. 1981. Post-Vietnam syndrome: Recognition and management. *Psychosomatics* 22: 931–42.

Friedman, R., and Gradstein, B. 1982. *Surviving pregnancy loss.* Boston: Little, Brown.

Froese, A., Hackett, T. P., Cassem, N. H., and Silverberg, E. L. 1974. Trajectories of anxiety and depression in denying and nondenying acute myocardial infarction patients during hospitalization. *J. Psychosomatic Res.* 18: 413–20.

Froese, A., Vasquez, E., Cassem, N. H., and Hackett, T. P. 1974. Validation of anxiety, depression and denial scales in a coronary care unit. *J. Psychosomatic Res.* 18: 137–41.

Fu, Y., Robboy, S. J., and Prat, J. 1978. Nuclear DNA study of vaginal and cervical squamous cell abnormalities in DES exposed progeny. *Ob. Gyn.* 52: 129–37.

Geschickter, C. F. 1939. Mammary carcinoma in the rat with metastasis induced by estrogen. *Science* 89: 35–37.

Gill, W. B., Schumacher, G. F. B., and Bibbo, M. 1976. Structural and functional abnormalities in the sex organs of male offspring of mothers treated with diethylstilbestrol (DES). *J. Reprod. Med.* 16: 147–53.

Gill, W. B., Schumacher, G. F. B., Bibbo, M., Straus, F. H., Schoenberg, H. W. 1979. Association of diethylstilbestrol exposure in utero with cryptorchidism, testicular hypoplasia and semen abnormalities. *J. Urology* 122: 36–39.

Gilligan, C. 1982. *In a different voice: Psychological theory and women's development.* Cambridge: Harvard University Press.

Gitman, L., and Koplowitz, A. 1950. Use of diethylstilbestrol in complications of pregnancy. *N.Y. State J. Med.* 50: 2823–2824.

Glauber, I. P. 1953. A deterrent in the study and practice of medicine. *Psychoanalytic Quarterly* 22: 381–412.

Glebatis, D. M., and Janerich, D. T. 1981. A statewide approach to diethylstilbestrol—the New York program. *New Eng. J. Med.* 304: 47–50.

Gold, J. J. 1975. *Gynecologic endocrinology.* Hagerstown, Md.: Harper and Row.

Greenwald, P., Barlow, J. J., Nasca, P. C., and Burnett, W. S. 1971. Vaginal cancer after maternal treatment with synthetic estrogens. *New Eng. J. Med.* 285: 390–92.

Greenwald, P., Nasca, P. C., Burnett, W. S., and Polan, A. 1973. Prenatal stilbestrol experience of mothers of young cancer patients. *Cancer* 31: 568–72.

Greer, A. L. 1977. Advances in the study of diffusion of innovation in health care organizations. *Milbank Mem. Fund. Q.: Health and Society* 55: 505–32.

Guttentag, O. E. 1953. The problem of experimentation on human beings: The physicians' point of view. *Science* 117: 207–10.

Hackett, T. P., and Cassem, N. H. 1974. Development of a quantitative rating scale to assess denial. *J. Psychosomatic Res.* 18: 93–100.

Hackett, T. P., Cassem, N. H., and Wishnie, H. A. 1968. The coronary care unit: An appraisal of its psychological hazards. *New Eng. J. Med.* 279: 1365–1370.

Haggerty, R. J. 1968. Diagnosis and treatment: Tonsils and adenoids—a problem revisited. *Pediatrics* 41: 815–17.

Hall, D. L. 1977. The social implications of the scientific study of sex. In *The scholar and the feminist IV: Connecting theory, practice and values.* The Women's Center, Barnard College, New York, N.Y. 10027. Brooklyn: Faculty Press, pp. 11–21.

Hammer, S. 1975. *Daughters and mothers, mothers and daughters.* New York: Quadrangle.

Hart, W. R., Townsend, D. E., Aldrich, J. O., Henderson, B. E., Roy, M., and Benton, B. 1976. Histopathologic spectrum of vaginal adenosis and related changes in stilbestrol-exposed females. *Cancer* 37: 763–75.

Hartman, M. S., and Banner, L. W. 1974. *Clio's consciousness raised: New perspectives on the history of women.* New York: Harper Colophon, Harper and Row.

Haseltine, F. P., and Ohno, S. 1981. Mechanisms of gonadal differentiation. *Science* 211: 1272–1278.

Hauser, S. T. 1981. Physician-patient relationships. In Mishler et al. 1981, pp. 104–40.

Heinonen, O. P. 1973. Diethylstilbestrol in pregnancy: Frequency of exposure and usage patterns. *Cancer* 31: 573–77.

Henderson, B. E., Benton, B., Cosgrove, M., Baptista, M. A., Aldrich, J., Townsend, D., Hart, W., and Mack, T. 1976. Urogenital tract abnormalities in sons of women treated with diethylstilbestrol. *Pediatrics* 58: 505–07.

Henderson, B. E., Benton, B., Jing, J., Yu, M. C., and Pike, M. C. 1979. Risk factors for cancer of the testis in young men. *Int. J. Cancer* 23: 598–602.

Hendricks, A. G., Benirschke, K., Thompson, R. S., Ahern, J. K., Lucas, W. E., Oi, R. H. 1979. The effects of prenatal diethylstilbestrol (DES) exposure on the genitalia of pubertal *macaca mulatta* I female offspring. *J. Reprod. Med.* 22: 233–40.

Hennig, M., and Jardim, A. 1978. *The managerial woman.* New York: Pocket Books.

Herbst, A. L., ed. 1978. *Intrauterine exposure to diethylstilbestrol in the human.* Proceedings of 1977 symposium on DES. American College of Obstetricians and Gynecologists.

Herbst, A. L. and Bern, H. A. 1981. *Developmental effects of diethylstilbestrol—(DES) in pregnancy.* New York: Thieme-Stratton.

Herbst, A. L., Cole, P., Cotton, T., Robboy, S. J., and Scully, R. E. 1977. Age-incidence and risk of diethylstilbestrol-related clear-cell adenocarcinoma of the vagina and cervix. *Am. J. Ob. Gyn.* 128: 43–50.

Herbst, A. L., Green, Jr., T. H., and Ulfelder, H. 1970. Primary carcinoma of the vagina. *Am. J. Ob. Gyn.* 106: 210–18.

Herbst, A. L., Hubby, M. M., Blough, R. R., and Azizi, F. 1980. A comparison of pregnancy experience in DES-exposed and DES-unexposed daughters. *J. Reprod. Med.* 24: 62–69.

Herbst, A., Kurman, R. J., and Scully, R. E. 1972. Vaginal and cervical abnormalities after exposure to stilbestrol *in utero. Ob. Gyn.* 40: 287–98.

Herbst, A. L., Poskanzer, D. C., Robboy, S. J., Friedlander, L., and Scully, R. E. 1975. Prenatal exposure to stilbestrol: A prospective comparison of exposed female offspring with unexposed controls. *New Eng. J. Med.* 292: 334–39.

Herbst, A. L., Robboy, S. J., MacDonald, G. J., and Scully, R. E. 1974. The effects of local progesterone on stilbestrol-associated vaginal adenosis. *Am. J. Ob. Gyn.* 118: 607–15.

Herbst, A. L., Robboy, S. J., Scully, R. E., and Poskanzer, D. C. 1974. Clear-cell adenocarcinoma of the vagina and cervix in girls: Analysis of 170 registry cases. *Am. J. Ob. Gyn.* 119: 713–24.

Herbst, A. L., and Scully, R. E. 1970. Adenocarcinoma of the vagina in adolescence: A report of 7 cases including 6 clear-cell carcinoma (so-called mesonephromas). *Cancer* 25: 745–57.

Herbst, A. L., Ulfelder, H., and Poskanzer, D. C. 1971. Adenocarcinoma of the vagina: Association of maternal stilbestrol therapy with tumor appearance in young women. *New Eng. J. Med.* 284: 878–81.

Hier, D. B., and Crowley, W. F. 1982. Spatial ability in androgen-deficient men. *New Eng. J. Med.* 306: 1202–1205.

Hippocrates. 1923. Loeb Classical Library, trans. W. H. S. Jones. 4 vols. Cambridge: Harvard University Press.

Hoefnagel, R. 1976. Prenatal diethylstilbestrol exposure and male hypogonadism. *Lancet* 17: 152–53.

Hoover, R., Gray, Sr., L. A., Fraumeni, Jr., J. F. 1977. Stilbestrol (diethylstilbestrol) and the risk of ovarian cancer. *Lancet* 2: 533–34.

Hoppe, K. 1971. The aftermath of Nazi persecution reflected in recent psychiatric literature. *Int. Psychiatry Clin.* 8: 169–204.

Horney, K. 1933. The denial of the vagina: A contribution to the problem of the genital anxieties specific to women. *Int. J. Psychoanalysis* 14: 55–70.

Hulka, B. S., Fowler, W. C., Kaufman, D. B., Grimson, R. C., Greenberg, B. G., Hogue, C. J. R., Berger, G. S., and Pulliam, C. C. 1980. Estrogen and endometrial cancer: Cases and two control groups from North Carolina. *Am. J. Ob. Gyn.* 137: 92–101.

Huntington, M. J. 1957. The development of a professional self-image. Pp. 179–187 in R. K. Newton *et al.* 1957.

Illich, I. 1975. *Medical nemesis: The expropriation of health.* New York: Bantam.

Jacobson, H. N., and Reid, D. E. 1964. High risk pregnancy: A pattern of comprehensive maternal and child care. *New Eng. J. Med.* 271: 302–07.

Johnson, L. D., Driscoll, S. G., Hertig, A. T., Cole, P. T., and Nickerson, R. J. 1979. Vaginal adenosis in stillborns and neonates exposed to diethylstilbestrol and steroidal estrogens and progestins. *Ob. Gyn.* 53: 671–79.

Johnson, L. D., Palmer, A. E., King, Jr., N. W., and Hertig, A. T. 1981. Vaginal adenosis in *cebus apella* monkeys exposed to DES in utero. *Ob. Gyn.* 57: 629–35.

Jones, L., and Tacillas-Verjan, R. 1979. Transplantability and sex steroid hormone responsiveness of cervico-vaginal tumors derived from BALP-cCrgl mice neonatally treated with ovarian steroids. *Cancer Res.* 39: 2591–2594.

Jordan, E. P. 1958. *Modern drug encyclopedia and therapeutic index.* 7th ed. New York: Drug Publications.

Journal of the American Medical Association. 1939. Estrogen therapy—a warning. *JAMA* 113: 2323–2324.

———. 1940. Contraindications to estrogen therapy. *JAMA* 114: 1560–1561.

———. 1979. Medical news: No DES for animal growth. *JAMA* 242: 1010.

Jukes, T. H. 1976. Diethylstilbestrol in beef production: What is the risk to consumers? *Prev. Med.* 5: 438–53.

Kalland, T., Rossberg, T. M., and Forsberg, J. 1978. Localization of ^{3}H-Estradiol-17beta in diethylstilbestrol-^{3}H induced adenosis. *Ob. Gyn.* 51: 464–67.

Kant, I. [1790]. 1951. *Critique of judgment.* New York: Hafner.

Karnaky, K. J. 1942. The use of stilbestrol for the treatment of threatened and habitual abortion and premature labor: A preliminary report. *Southern Med. J.* 35: 838–47.

Katz, J. 1972. *Experimentation with human beings.* New York: Russell Sage.

Kaufman, R. H., Adam, E., Binder, G. L., and Gerthoffer, E. 1980. Upper genital tract changes and pregnancy outcome in offspring exposed in utero to diethylstilbestrol. *Am. J. Ob. Gyn.* 137: 299–308.

Kaufman, R. H., Binder, G. L., Gray, Jr., P. M., and Adam, E. 1977. Upper genital tract changes associated with exposure in utero to diethylstilbestrol. *Am. J. Ob. Gyn.* 128: 51–59.

Kijak, M., and Funtowicz, S. 1982. The syndrome of the survivor of extreme situations. *Int. Rev. Psycho-anal.* 9: 25–33.

King. A. G. 1953. Threatened and repeated abortion: Present status of therapy. *Ob. Gyn.* 1: 104–14.

Kinston, W., and Rosser, R. 1974. Disaster: Effects on mental and physical state. *J. Psychosomatic Res.* 18: 437–56.

Kirkpatrick, M. 1980. *Women's sexual development: Exploration of inner space.* New York: Plenum Press.

Kistner, R. W. 1976. Can young women with vaginal or cervical adenosis take oral contraceptives? *JAMA* 235: 2536.

Knowles, J. H., ed. 1968. *Views of medical education and medical care.* Cambridge: Harvard University Press.

Knox, R. A. 1980. For "DES daughters," a study finds a note of reassurance. *Boston Globe,* August 1, p. 1.

Krakowski, A. J. 1979. Liaison psychiatry: A service for averting dehumanization of medicine. *Psychother. Psychosom.* 32: 164–69.

Krill, C. E., and Toomey, J. A. 1941. Multiple cases of tonsillectomy and poliomyelitis. *JAMA* 117: 1013–17.

Kurzrok, R., Kitson, L., and Perloff, W. H. 1940. The action of diethylstilbestrol in gynecological dysfunctions. *Endocrinology* 26: 581–86.

Labarthe, D., Adam, E., Noller, K., O'Brien, P. C., Robboy, S. J., Tilley, B. S., Townsend, D., Barnes, A. B., Kaufman, R. H., Decker, D. G., Fish, C. R., Herbst, A. L., Gunderson, J., and Kurland, L. T. 1978. Design and preliminary observations of national cooperative diethylstilbestrol adenosis project. *Ob. Gyn.* 51: 453–58.

Lacassagne, A. 1938. Apparition d'adénocarcinomes mammaires chez des souris males traitées par une substance oestrogène synthétique [Appearance of mammary adenocarcinoma in male mice treated with a synthetic estrogenic substance]. *Comptes rendu des séances de la Société de Biologie* 129: 641–43.

Lain Entralgo, P. 1969. *Doctor and patient.* New York: McGraw-Hill.

Langebartel, D. A. 1929. *The anatomical primer: An embryological explanation of human gross morphology.* Baltimore: University Park Press.

Lanier, A. P., Noller, K. L., Decker, D. G., Elveback, L. R., and Kurland, L. T. 1973. Cancer and stilbestrol: A follow-up of 1,719 persons exposed to estrogens in utero and born 1943–1959. *Mayo Clin. Proc.* 48: 793–99.

Lasagna, L. 1982. Historical controls: The practitioner's clinical trials. *New Eng. J. Med.* 307: 1339–1340.

Lazare, A., and Eisenthal, S. 1977. Patient requests in a walk-in clinic. *J. Nervous and Mental Disease* 165: 330–40.

Lazare, A., Eisenthal, S., and Wasserman, L. 1975. The customer approach to patienthood: Attending to patient requests in a walk-in clinic. *Arch. Gen. Psychiatry* 32: 553–58.

Lederer, W. 1968. *The fear of women.* New York: Harvest Books.

Lerner, H. E. 1974. Early origins of envy and devaluation of women. *Bull. Menninger Clinic* 38: 538–53.

Levi, P. 1959. *Survival in Auschwitz.* New York: Orion Press.

Lieberman, M., and Tobin, S. 1983. *The experience of old age: Stress, coping and survival.* In *Personality and adaptation,* pp. 172–202. New York: Basic.

Lifton, R. J. 1963. Psychological effects of the atomic bomb in Hiroshima: The theme of death. *Daedalus* 92: 462–97.

Lilienfeld, A. 1982. Ceteris paribus: The evolution of the clinical trial. *Bull. Hist. Med.* 56: 1–18.

Lindemann, E. 1944. Symptomatology and management of acute grief. *Am. J. Psychiatry* 101: 141–48.

Linden, G., and Henderson, B. E. 1972. Genital-tract cancers in adolescents and young adults. *New Eng. J. Med.* 286: 760–61.

Loeb, L. 1919. Further investigations on the origin of tumors in mice: Internal secretion as a factor in the origin of tumors. *J. Med. Res.* 40: 477ff.

Loeb, L. 1935. Estrogenic hormones and carcinogenesis. In *Glandular physiology and therapy,* pp. 177–92. Chicago. American Medical Association.

Loeb, L., Burns, E. L., Suntzeff, V., and Moskop, M. 1936. Carcinoma-like proliferations in vagina, cervix and the uterus of mouse treated with estrogenic hormones. *Proc. Soc. Exper. Biol. Med.* 35: 320–22.

Love, S. M., Gelman, R. S., and Silen, W. 1982. Fibrocystic disease of the breast—a non-disease? *New Eng. J. Med.* 307: 1010–1014.

Lyden, F. J., Geiger, H. J., and Peterson, O. L. 1968. *The training of good physicians: Critical factors in career choices.* Cambridge: Harvard University Press.

MacBride, C. M., Freedman, H., and Loeffel, E. 1939. Studies on stilbestrol: Preliminary statement. *JAMA* 113: 2320–2323.

McCarthy, E., Finkel, M. L., and Ruchlin, H. S. 1981. *Second opinion elective surgery.* Boston: Auburn House.

McKinlay, J. B. 1981. From "promising report" to "standard procedure": Seven stages in the career of a medical innovation. *Milbank Mem. Fund. Q.: Health and Society* 59: 374–411.

McLachlan, J. A., Newbold, R. R., and Bullock, B. 1975. Reproductive tract lesions in male mice exposed prenatally to diethylstilbestrol. *Science* 190: 991–92.

———. 1980. Long-term effects on the female mouse genital tract associated with prenatal exposure to diethylstilbestrol. *Cancer Res.* 40: 3988–3999.

MacMahon, B., Pugh, T. F., and Ipsen, J. 1960. *Epidemiologic methods.* Boston: Little, Brown.

Mahler, H. 1977. Problems of medical affluence. *WHO Chronicle* 31: 8–13.

Maloney, M. J., and Klykylo, W. M. 1983. An overview of anorexia nervosa, bulimia and obesity in children and adolescents. *J. Am. Acad. Child Psych.* 22: 99–107.

Mann, E. C. 1956. Psychiatric investigation of habitual abortion—preliminary report. *Ob. Gyn.* 7: 589–601.

———. 1959. Habitual abortion: A report in 2 parts on 160 patients. *Am. J. Ob. Gyn.* 77: 706–18.

Mattingly, R. F., and Stafl, A. 1976. Cancer risk in diethylstilbestrol-exposed offspring. *Am. J. Ob. Gyn.* 126: 543–48.

Merck Index. 1960. Ed. Paul G. Stecher. 7th ed. Rahway, N.J.: Merck.

Meyer-Bahlburg, H. F. L. 1978. Behavioral effects of estrogen treatments in human males. *Pediatrics* 62 (supplement, part 2): 1171–1177.

Meyers, R. 1983. *DES—the bitter pill.* New York: Seaview/Putnam.

Millman, M. 1977. *The unkindest cut: Life in the backrooms of medicine.* New York: William Morrow.

Mills, J. L., and Bongiovanni, A. M. 1978. Effect of prenatal estrogen exposure on male genitalia. *Pediatrics* 62 (supplement, part 2): 1160–1164.

Mink, Patsy Takemoto *et al.* v. University of Chicago *et al.* 1982. Depositions and transcripts of trial, no. 77 C 1431 before Judge John F. Grady in the United States District Court for the Northeastern District of Illinois, Eastern Division. 460 F. Supp. 713 (N.D. ILL. 1978) and 27 F.R. Serv 2D. 739 (N.D. ILL. 1979).

Mishler, E. G. 1979. Meaning in context: Is there any other kind? *Harvard Ed. Rev.* 49: 1–19.

———. 1982. The discourse of medicine: Dialectics of medical interviews. Revised manuscript.

Mishler, E. G., Amara, S. L. R., Hauser, S. T., Liem, R., Osherson, S. D., and Waxler, N. E. 1981. *Social contexts of health, illness and patient care.* Cambridge: Cambridge University Press.

Monaghan, J. M., and Sirisena, L. A. W. 1978. Stilboestrol and vaginal clear-cell adenocarcinoma syndrome. *Brit. Med. J.* 1: 1588–1590.

Money, J., and Ehrhardt, A. A. 1972a. Gender dimorphic behavior and fetal sex hormones. *Recent Prog. Horm. Res.* 28: 735–63.

———. 1972b. *Man and woman: Boy and girl.* Baltimore: Johns Hopkins University Press.

Money, J., Hampson, J. G., and Hampson, J. L. 1957. Imprinting and the establishment of gender role. *Arch. Neurol. Psych.* 77: 333–36.

Morantz, R. 1974. The lady and her physician. In Hartman and Banner, 1974.

Morrell, J. A. 1941. Summary of some clinical reports on stilbestrol. *J. Clin. Endocrinology* 1: 419–23.

Morrow, C. P., and Townsend, D. E. 1975. Management of adenosis and clear-cell adenocarcinoma of vagina and cervix. *J. Reprod. Med.* 15: 25–28.

Moulton, R. 1977. Some effects of the new feminism. *Am. J. Psychiatry* 134: 1–6.

Ms. Magazine. 1983. N. Zamichow, "Is it something in the food? The mystery of the frightful epidemic of early sexual development." Vol. 12, no. 4 (December): 92–94, 141–43.

Mucklé, C. W. 1940. The suppression of lactation by stilbestrol. *Am. J. Ob. Gyn.* 40: 133–35.

Nadelson, C. C., and Notman, M. T. 1982. *The woman patient.* Vol. 2, *Concepts of femininity and the Life Cycle.* New York: Plenum Press.

Nadelson, C. C., Notman, M. T., Miller, J. B., and Zilbach, J. 1982. Aggression in women: Conceptual issues and clinical implications. In *The woman patient;* Vol. 3, *Aggression, adaptations and psychotherapy,* ed. M. T. Notman and C. C. Nadelson. New York: Plenum, 1978.

Naftolin, F., and Butz, E., eds. 1981. *Sexual dimorphism. Science* 211, no. 4488 (20 March): complete issue.

Naftulin, D. H., Ware, J. E., and Donnelly, F. A. 1973. The Doctor Fox lecture: A paradigm of educational seduction. *J. Med. Educ.* 48: 630–35.

National Cancer Institute (NCI). 1981a. Were you or your daughter or son born after 1940? An important message from the U.S. Public Health Service. NIH publication no. 81–1226. (This and other NCI publications are available free from Office of Cancer Communications, NCI, Room 10A17, National Institutes of Health, Bethesda, Md. 20014.)

———. 1981b. Questions and answers about DES exposure during pregnancy and before birth. NIH. publication no. 81–1118.

————. 1981c. Prenatal diethylstilbestrol (DES) exposure: Recommendations of the Diethylstilbestrol-Adenosis (DESAD) project for the identification and management of exposed individuals. NIH publication no. 81–2049.

Neumann, E. 1963. *The great mother: An analysis of the archetype.* New York: Pantheon.

New, M. I., Levine, L. S., Yaffee, S. J., Soyka, L. I., Gurpide, E., Segal, S. J., and Van Wyck, J. J. 1978. Report of the conference on estrogen treatment of the young. *Pediatrics* 62 (part 2): 1087–1217.

Newbold, R. R., Bullock, B. C., and McLachlan, J. A. 1983. Diethylstilbestrol during pregnancy permanently alters the ovary and oviduct. *Biol. Reproduction* 28: 735–44.

Newbold, R. R., and McLachlan, J. A. 1981. Vaginal adenosis and adenocarcinoma in mice exposed transplacentally to diethylstilbestrol. *Cancer Res.* 42: 2003–2011.

Newbold, R. R., Tyrey, S., Haney, A. F., and McLachlan, J. A. 1983. Developmentally arrested oviduct: A structural and functional deficit in mice following pre-natal exposure to diethylstilbestrol. *Teratology* 27: 417–26.

Newman, C. J. 1976. Children of disaster: Clinical observations at Buffalo Creek. *Am. J. Psychiatry* 133: 306–12.

Newton, M. 1973. Editorial about ACOG Technical Bulletin on DES, encouraging casefinding. *ACOG Newsletter* 17(5): 2.

Newton, N. 1955. *A study of women's feelings toward menstruation, pregnancy, childbirth, breastfeeding, infant care and other aspects of their femininity.* Psychosomatic Medicine Monographs. New York: Hoeber, Harper and Bros.

Newton, R. K., Reader, G., and Kendall, P. L. eds. 1957. *The student physician.* Cambridge: Harvard University Press.

Ng, A. B., Reagan, J. W., Nadji, M., and Greening, S. 1977. Natural history of vaginal adenosis in women exposed to diethylstilbestrol *in utero. J. Reprod. Med.* 18: 1–13.

Niederland, W. G. 1974. *The Schreber case.* New York: Quadrangle Press.

Nissen, E. D., and Goldstein, A. I. 1973. Stilbestrol therapy in pregnancy. *Int. J. Gyn. Ob.* 11: 133–42.

Noller, K. L., Townsend, D. E., Kaufman, B. H., Barnes, A. B., Robboy, S. J., Fish, C. R., Jeffries, J. A., Bergstralh, E. J., O'Brien, P. C., McGorray, S., and Scully, R. 1983. Maturation of vaginal and cervical epithelium in women exposed in utero to diethylstilbestrol. DESAD project. *Am. J. Ob. Gyn.* 146: 279–85.

Notman, M. T., and Nadelson, C. C. 1978. *The woman patient.* Vol. 1, *Sexual and reproductive aspects of women's health care.* New York: Plenum.

Novak, E., and Woodruff, J. D., eds. 1979. *Novak's gynecologic and obstetric pathology with clinical and endocrine relation.* 8th ed. Philadelphia: Saunders.

Nunley, W. C., and Kitchin, J. D. 1979. Successful management of incompetent cervix in a primigravida exposed to diethylstilbestrol in utero. *Fertility and Sterility* 31: 217–19.

Orenberg, C. L. 1981. *DES: The complete story.* New York: St. Martin's.

Osmond, H. 1980. God and the doctor. *New Eng. J. Med.* 302: 555–58.

Paget, M. A. 1978. *The unity of mistakes: A phenomenological study of medical work.* Ph.D. diss., Michigan State University.

Payne, F. L., and Mucklé, C. W. 1940. Stilbestrol in the treatment of menopausal symptoms. *Am. J. Ob. Gyn.* 40: 135–39.

Peabody, F. W. 1927. The care of the patient. *JAMA* 88: 878–82.

Pearson, W., and Clark, M. 1982. The mal(e) treatment of American women in gynecology and obstetrics. *Int. J. Women's Studies* 5: 338–47.

Pederson, P. M. 1947. A statistical study of poliomyelitis in relationship to tonsillectomy. *Annals of Otolaryngology, Rhinology, Laryngology* 56: 1281–1293.

Peña, E. F. 1954. Prevention of abortion. *Am. J. Surg.* 87: 95–96.

Perl, M., and Shelp, E. 1982. Psychiatric consultation masking moral dilemmas in medicine. *New Eng. J. Med.* 307: 618–21.

Peterson, O. 1956. An analytic study of North Carolina general practice 1953–54. *J. Med. Educ.* 31, part 2.

Physicians' Desk Reference 1947–83. 37 editions. Oradell, N.J.: Medical Economics Co.

Pietras, R. J., Szego, C. M., Mangan, C. E., Seeler, B. J., Burtnett, M. M., and Orevi, M. 1978. Elevated serum cathepsin B1 and vaginal pathology after prenatal DES exposure. *Ob. Gyn.* 52: 321–27.

Plate, W. P. 1954. Diethylstilbestrol therapy in habitual abortion. *Proc. Int. Cong. Ob. Gyn. Geneva:* 751–57.

Pomerance, W. 1973. Post-stilbestrol secondary syndrome. *Ob. Gyn.* 42: 12–18.

Popper, K. R. 1962. *Conjectures and refutations: The growth of scientific knowledge.* New York: Basic.

Poskanzer, D. C., and Herbst, A. L. 1977. Epidemiology of vaginal adenosis and adenocarcinoma associated with exposure to stilbestrol *in utero. Cancer* 39: 1892–1895.

Prins, R. P., Morrow, C. P., Townsend, D. E., and Disaia, P. J. 1976. Vaginal embryogenesis, estrogens and adenosis. *Ob. Gyn.* 48: 246–50.

Putnam, J. J. 1899. *Not the disease only, but also the man.* Boston: Shattuck Lecture.

Quigley, M. M., and Hammond, C. B. 1979. Estrogen-replacement therapy—help or hazard? *New Eng. J. Med.* 301: 646–48.

Rabin, D. 1982. Compounding the ordeal of ALS: Isolation from my fellow physicians. *New Eng. J. Med.* 307: 506–09.

Ramsey, P. 1970. *The patient as a person.* New Haven: Yale University Press.

———. 1975. *The ethics of fetal research.* New Haven: Yale University Press.

Randall, C. L., Baetz, R. W., Hall, D. W., and Birtch, P. K. 1955. Pregnancies observed in the likely-to-abort patient with or without hormone therapy before or after conception. *Am. J. Ob. Gyn.* 69: 643–56.

Rangell, L. 1976. Discussion of the Buffalo Creek disaster: The course of psychic trauma. *Am. J. Psychiatry* 133: 313–16.

Reddoch, J. W., and Wiener, W. B. 1943. Stilbestrol in the termination of pregnancy. *Am. J. Ob. Gyn.* 45: 343–47.

Reid, D. D. 1955. Use of hormones in the management of pregnancy in diabetes. *Lancet* 2: 833–36.

Reinisch, J. M. 1974. Fetal hormones, the brain and human sex differences: A heuristic, integrative review of the literature. *Arch. Sexual Behavior* 3: 51–90.

Reinisch, J. M., and Karow, W. C. 1977. Prenatal exposure to synthetic progestins and estrogens: Effects on human development. *Arch. Sexual Behavior* 6: 257–88.

Relman, A. S. 1980. Here come the women (editorial). *New Eng. J. Med.* 302: 1252–1253.

Rennell, C. L. 1979. T-shaped uterus in diethylstilbestrol (DES) exposure. *Am. J. Roentgenology* 132: 979–80.

Richart, R. M., Townsend, D. E., Crisp, W., DePetrillo, A., Ferenczy, A., Johnson, G., Lickrish, G., Roy, M., Villasanta, U. 1980. An analysis of "long-term" follow-up results in patients with cervical intraepithelial neoplasia treated by cryotherapy *Am. J. Ob. Gyn.* 137: 823–26.

Richmond, J. 1978. Physician advisory: Health effects of the pregnancy use of diethylstilbestrol. Surgeon-General's advisory sent to physicians, 4 October 1978. Published in 1979 in *Clinical Toxicology* 14: 313–18.

Robboy, S. J., Friedlander, L. M., Welch, W. R., Keh, P., Taft, P. D., Barnes, A. B., Scully, R. E., and Herbst, A. L. 1976. Cytology of 575 young women with prenatal exposure to diethylstilbestrol. *Ob. Gyn.* 48: 511–15.

Robboy, S. J., Herbst, A. L., and Scully, R. E. 1974. Clear-cell adenocarcinoma of the vagina and cervix in young women: Analysis of 37 tumors that persisted or recurred after primary therapy. *Cancer* 34: 606–14.

Robboy, S. J., Keh, P. C., Nickerson, R. J., Helmanis, E. K., Prat, J., Szyfelbein, W. M., Taft, P. D., Barnes, A. B., Scully, R. E., and Welch, W. R. 1978. Squamous cell dysplasia and carcinoma in situ of the cervix and vagina after prenatal exposure to diethylstilbestrol. *Ob. Gyn.* 51: 529–35.

Robboy, S. J., Prat, J., Welch, W. R., and Barnes, A. B. 1977. Squamous cell neoplasia controversy in the female exposed to diethylstilbestrol. *Human Pathol.* 8: 483–85.

Robboy, S. J., Scully, R. E., and Herbst, A. L. 1975. Pathology of vaginal and cervical abnormalities associated with prenatal exposure to diethylstilbestrol (DES). *J. Reprod. Med.* 15: 13–18.

Robboy, S. J., Szyfelbein, W. M., Goellner, J. R., Kaufman, R. H., Taft, P. D., Richard, R. M., Gaffey, T. A., Prat, J., Virata, R., Hatab, P. A., McGorray, S. P., Noller, K. L., Townsend, D., Labarthe, D., and Barnes, A. B. 1981. Dysplasia and cytologic findings in 4,589 young women enrolled in Diethylstilbestrol-Adenosis (DESAD) project. *Am. J. Ob. Gyn.* 140: 579–86.

Robboy, S. J., and Welch, W. R. 1977. Microglandular hyperplasia in vaginal adenosis associated with oral contraceptives and prenatal diethylstilbestrol exposure. *Ob. Gyn.* 49: 430–34.

Robboy, S. J., Young, R. H., and Herbst, A. 1982. Female genital tract changes related to prenatal diethylstilbestrol exposure. Chap. 4 In *Pathology of the female genital tract,* ed. A. Blaustein, 2d ed. New York: Springer-Verlag.

Robinson, D., and Shettles, L. B. 1952. The use of diethylstilbestrol in threatened abortion. *Am. J. Ob. Gyn.* 63: 1330–1333.

Roiphe, H., and Galenson, E. 1982. *Infantile origins of sexual identity.* New York: International Universities Press.

Romney, S. L., Gray, M. J., Little, A. B., Merrill, J., Quilligan, E. J., and

Stander, R. W. 1981. *Gynecology and obstetrics: The health care of women.* 2d ed. New York: McGraw-Hill.

Rosenberg, L., Shapiro, S., Kaufman, D. W., Slone, D., Miettinen, O. S., and Stolley, P. D. 1979. Patterns and determinants of conjugated estrogen use. *Am. J. Epidemiology* 109: 676–86.

Rosenfeld, D. L., and Bronson, R. A. 1980. Reproductive problems in the DES-exposed female. *Ob. Gyn.* 55: 453–56.

Ross, J. W. 1953. Further report on the use of diethylstilbestrol in the treatment of threatened abortion. *J. Nat. Med. Assoc.* 45: 223ff.

Rourk, Jr., M. H., Hock, R. A., Pursell, J. S., Jones, D., and Spock, A. 1981. The news media and the doctor-patient relationship. *New Eng. J. Med.* 305: 1278–1280.

Russ, J. S., and Collins, C. G. 1940. The treatment of prepubertal vulvovaginitis with a new synthetic estrogen. *JAMA* 114: 2446–2450.

Ruzek, S. B., ed. 1978. *The women's health movement: Feminist alternatives to medical control.* New York: Praeger.

Ryan, K. J. 1978. Diethylstilbestrol: Twenty-five years later. Editorial. *New Eng. J. Med.* 298: 794–95.

Sackett, D. L. 1975. Design, measurement and analysis in clinical trials. In *Platelets, drugs and thrombosis,* J. Hirsch. Basel: Karger.

Sacks, H., Chalmers, T. C., and Smith, Jr., H. 1982. Randomized versus historical controls for clinical trials. *Am. J. Med.* 72: 238–40.

Sandberg, E. C. 1968. The incidence and distribution of occult vaginal adenosis. *Am. J. Ob. Gyn.* 101: 1322–1324.

———. 1976. Benign cervical and vaginal changes associated with exposure to stilbestrol in utero. *Am. J. Ob. Gyn.* 125: 777–89.

Sandberg, E. C., and Christian, J. C. 1980. Diethylstilbestrol-exposed monozygotic twins discordant for cervicovaginal clear-cell adenocarcinoma. *Am. J. Ob. Gyn.* 137: 220–28.

Sandberg, E. C., Danielson, R. W., Cauwet, R. W., and Bonar, B. F. 1965. Adenosis vaginae. *Am. J. Ob. Gyn.* 93: 209–22.

Sandberg, E. C., Riffle, N. L., Higdon, J. V., and Getman, C. 1981. Pregnancy outcome in women exposed to diethylstilbestrol in utero. *Am. J. Ob. Gyn.* 140: 194–205.

Schmidt, G., and Fowler, Jr., W. C. 1980. Cervical stenosis following minor gynecologic procedures on DES-exposed women. *Ob. Gyn.* 56: 333–35.

Schmidt, G., Fowler, Jr., W. C., Talbert, L. M., and Edelman, D. A. 1980. Reproductive history of women exposed to diethylstilbestrol in utero. *Fertility and Sterility* 33: 21–24.

Schmitt, A. W. 1976. Moderator, Management of the DES syndrome, clear-cell carcinoma excluded: A discussion. *J. Reprod. Med.* 16(6): 282–98.

Schowalter, J. E. 1977. The adolescent with cancer. In *The experience of dying,* ed. E. M. Pattison. Englewood Cliffs, N.J.: Prentice-Hall.

———. 1983a. The psyche and soma of physical illness in adolescence. *Psychosomatics* 24: 453–61.

———. 1983b. Mood disturbance in physical illness in adolescence. In *The adolescent and mood disturbance,* ed. H. Golombek and B. D. Barfinkel. New York: International Universities Press.

Schwartz, R. W., and Stewart, N. B. 1977. Psychological effects of DES exposure. *JAMA* 237: 252–54.

Science. 1979. Surgeon General seeks physicians' help in DES alert. *Science* 203: 159.

Scott, J. W., Seckinger, D., and Puente-Duany, E. 1974. Colposcopic aspects of management of vaginal adenosis in DES children. *J. Reprod. Med.* 12: 187–93.

Scully, R. E., Robboy, S. J., and Herbst, A. L. 1974. Vaginal and cervical abnormalities including clear-cell adenocarcinoma, related to prenatal exposure to stilbestrol. *Ann. Clin. Lab. Sci.* 4: 222–33.

Seaman, B., and Seaman, G. 1978. *Women and the crisis in sex hormones.* New York: Bantam.

Seibel, M., and Graves, W. L. 1980. The psychological implications of spontaneous abortions. *J. Reprod. Med.* 25: 161–65.

Seibel, M., and Taymor, M. L. 1982. Emotional aspects of infertility. *Fertility and Sterility* 37: 137–45.

Semmelweis, I. P. 1861 [1941]. The etiology, the concept and the prophylaxis of childbed fever. Trans. F. P. Murphy. *Med. Classics* 5: 350–773.

Semmelweis, I. P. 1972. Entry in *Encyclopedia Britannica* 20: 212–13.

Sestili, M. A. 1977. Brief report on the DESAD project: Genital tract abnormalities and cancer in females exposed in utero to diethylstilbestrol. *Public Health Reports,* September–October.

Sevringhaus, E. L. 1938. *Endocrine therapy in general practice.* 1st ed. Chicago: Yearbook Publications.

———. 1939. A woman faces fifty. *Hygieia* 17: 685–88, 752–53.

Shapiro, S., and Slone, D. 1979. The effects of exogenous female hormones on the fetus. In *Epidemiologic Review,* vol. 1, ed. P. E. Sartwell, pp. 110–23. Baltimore: Johns Hopkins University Press.

Shaw, N. S. 1974. *Forced labor: Maternity care in the United States.* Elmsford, N.Y.: Pergamon Press.

Sherman, A. I., Goldrath, M., Berlin, A., Vakhariya, V., Banooni, F., Michaels, W., Goodman, P., and Brown, J. 1974. Cervical-vaginal adenosis after *in-utero* exposure to synthetic estrogens. *Ob. Gyn.* 44: 531–45.

Shimkin, M. B., and Grady, H. G. 1940. Carcinogenic potency of stilbestrol and estrone in strain C_3H mice. *J. NCI* 1: 119–28.

Shopper, M. 1980. Psycho-analysis of a DES daughter. Unpublished paper presented during a panel of the American Academy of Child Psychiatry, "DES—A Paradigm of Modern Drug Abuse," Chicago, Ill., 18 October 1980.

Shorr, E., Robinson, F. N., and Papanicolaou, G. N. 1939. A clinical study of the synthetic estrogen stilbestrol. *JAMA* 113: 2312–2318.

Siders, D. B., Parrott, M. H., and Abell, M. R. 1965. Gland cell prosoplasia (adenosis) of vagina. *Am. J. Ob. Gyn.* 93: 190–203.

Silverman, W. A. 1980a. *Retrolental fibroplasia: A modern parable.* New York: Grune and Stratton.

———. 1980b. Medical inflation. *Perspect. Biol. Med.* 23: 617–37.

———. 1980c. Limitations of observational data. *Proc. Royal College Ob. Gyn.* (London): 293–306.

Simmel, E. 1926. The doctor-game, illness and the profession of medicine. *Int. J. Psycho-Anal.* 7: 470–83. Also in *The psycho-analytic reader,* ed. R. Fliess. 1948. New York: International Universities Press, pp. 259–72.

Simon, B. 1978. *Mind and madness in ancient Greece: The classical roots of modern psychiatry.* Ithaca, N.Y.: Cornell University Press.

Sinaiko, H. L. 1965. *Love, knowledge, and discourse in Plato: Dialogue and dialectic in Phaedrus, Republic, Parmenides.* Chicago: University of Chicago Press.

Singer, P. 1976. "Bioethics": The case of the fetus. *N.Y. Rev. Books,* 5 August.

Sipe, P. 1982. The wonder drug we should wonder about. *Science for the People,* November–December, pp. 9–33.

Skinner, C. O. 1955. Address to the American Gynecological Society. In *Bottoms Up!* New York: Dodd, Mead, pp. 199–208.

Smith, G. V., and Smith, O. W. 1941. Estrogen and progestin metabolism in pregnancy: The effect of hormone administration in pre-eclampsia. *J. Clin. Endocrinology* 1: 477–84.

———. 1944a. Pituitary stimulating property of stilbestrol as compared with that of estrone. *Proc. Soc. Exper. Bio. Med.* 57: 198–200.

————. 1944b. Pituitary studies of mature male rats' responses to an oxidative inactivation product of estrone. *Endocrinology* 35: 146–47.

————. 1945. Further studies of pituitary responses to an oxidative inactivation product of estrone. *Proc. Soc. Exper. Biol. Med.* 59: 242–46.

————. 1946. Increased excretion of pregnanediol in pregnancy from diethylstilbestrol with special reference to the prevention of late pregnancy accidents. *Am. J. Ob. Gyn.* 51: 411–15.

————. 1947a. Late pregnancy toxemia: A review of experimental findings. *Western J. Ob. Gyn.* 55: 288–94.

————. 1947b. Late pregnancy toxemia: Clinical trials based on experimental findings. *Western J. Ob. Gyn.* 55: 313–22.

————. 1948. Internal secretions and toxemia of late pregnancy. *Physiol. Rev.* 28: 1–22.

————. 1949a. The influence of diethylstilbestrol on the progress and outcome of pregnancy as based on a comparison of treated with untreated primigravidas. *Am. J. Ob. Gyn.* 58: 994–1009.

————. 1949b. The prophylactic use of diethylstilbestrol to prevent fetal loss from complications of late pregnancy. *New Eng. J. Med.* 241: 410–12.

————. 1950a. Does the excretion of diethylstilbestrol glucuronide influence the Venning determination of urinary pregnandediol? *Proc. Soc. Exper. Biol. Med.* 73: 378–81.

————. 1950b. The quantitative determination of urinary pregnanediol: Influence of method upon results. *J. Clin. Endocrinology* 10: 496–510.

————. 1952. Factors influencing the composition of the sodium "pregnanediol" glucuronide complex in human pregnancy with special reference to stilbestrol therapy. *J. Clin. Endocr. Met.* 12: 151–68.

————. 1953. Clinical results with stilbestrol in pregnancy. *Trans. New Eng. Ob. Gyn. Soc.* 7: 155–61.

————. 1954. Prophylactic hormone therapy: relation to complications of pregnancy. *Ob. Gyn.* 4: 129–41.

Smith, O. W. 1948. Diethylstilbestrol in the prevention and treatment of complications of pregnancy. *Am. J. Ob. Gyn.* 56: 821–34.

Smith, O. W., and Vanderlinde, R. E. 1951. An oxidative inactivation product of stilbestrol: Effects upon the rat pituitary. *Endocrinology* 49: 742–54.

Smithells, R. W. 1975. Iatrogenic hazards and their effects. *Postgrad. Med. J.* 15: 39–52.

Smith-Rosenberg, C. 1974. Puberty to menopause: The cycle of femininity in nineteenth century America. In *Clio's consciousness raised,* Mary S. Hartman and L. W. Banner. New York: Harper and Row, pp. 12–37.

Smith-Rosenberg, C., and Rosenberg, C. 1973. The female animal: Medical and biological views of women and her role in nineteenth century America. *J. Am. Hist.* 60: 332–56.

Sommers, S. C., Lawley, T. B., and Hertig, A. T. 1949. A study of the placenta in pregnancy treated by stilbestrol. *Am. J. Ob. Gyn.* 58: 1010–1013.

Spiro, H. M. 1975. Myths and mirths—women in medicine. *New Eng. J. Med.* 292: 354–56.

Spitz, R. A. 1952. Authority and masturbation. *Psychoanalytic Q.* 21: 490–527.

Stafl, A. 1975. Clinical detection of vaginal adenosis and clear-cell adenocarcinoma. *J. Reprod. Med.* 15: 19–24.

Stafl, A., Mattingly, R. F. 1974. Vaginal adenosis: A precancerous lesion? *Am. J. Ob. Gyn.* 120: 666–77.

Stafl, A., Mattingly, R. F., Foley, D. V., and Fetherston, W. C. 1974. Clinical diagnosis of vaginal adenosis. *Ob. Gyn.* 43: 118–28.

Starr, P. 1983. *The social transformation of American medicine.* New York: Basic.

Stern, G. M. 1976. From chaos to responsibility. *Am. J. Psychiatry* 133: 300–01.

Stillman, R. J. 1982. *In utero* exposure to diethylstilbestrol: Adverse effects on the reproductive tract and reproductive performance in mother and female offspring. *Am. J. Ob. Gyn.* 142: 905–21.

Stoller, R. J. 1979. A contribution to the study of gender identity. *Int. J. Psycho-analysis* 60: 433–41.

Sugar, M., ed. 1979. *Female adolescent development.* New York: Brunner/Mazel.

Sutherland, S., and Scherl, D. 1970. Patterns of response among victims of rape. *Am. J. Orthopsychiatry* 40: 503–11.

Swyer, G. I. M., and Law, R. G. 1954. An evaluation of the prophylactic antenatal use of stilboestrol: Preliminary report. *J. Endocrinology* 10: vi–vii.

Taft, P. D., Robboy, S. J., Herbst, A. L., and Scully, R. E. 1974. Cytology of clear-cell adenocarcinoma of genital tract in young females: Review of 95 cases from the registry. *Acta Cytol.* 18: 279–90.

Taussig, H. B. 1963. The evils of camouflage as illustrated by Thalidomide. *New Eng. J. Med.* 269: 92–94.

Temin, P. 1980. *Taking your medicine: Drug regulation in the U.S.* Cambridge: Harvard University Press.

Terr, L. C. 1979. Children of Chowchilla. *Psychoanalytic Study of the Child* 34: 547–627.

———. 1981a. Forbidden games. *J. Am. Acad. Child Psychiatry* 20: 741–60.

———. 1981b. Psychic trauma in children: Observations following the Chowchilla school-bus kidnapping. *Am. J. Psychiatry* 138: 14–19.

———. 1983a. Life attitudes, dreams and psychic trauma in a group of "normal" children. *J. Am. Acad. Child Psychiatry* 22: 221–30.

———. 1983b. Chowchilla revisited: The effects of psychic trauma four years after a school-bus kidnapping. *Am. J. Psychiatry* 140: 1543–1550.

Thiam, A. 1983. Women's fight for the abolition of sexual mutilation. *Int. Soc. Sci. J.* 35: 747–56.

Thompson, M. 1949. *The cry and the covenant.* Garden City, N.Y.: Doubleday.

Thucydides. 1951. *The Peloponnesian War.* Trans. Crawley. Modern Library edition. New York: Random House.

Titchener, J. L., and Kapp, F. T. 1976. Family and character change at Buffalo Creek. *Am. J. Psychiatry* 133: 295–99.

Tsukada, Y., Hewett, W. J., Barlow, J. J., and Pickren, J. W. Clear-cell adenocarcinoma (mesonephroma) of the vagina. *Cancer* 29: 1208–1214.

Tyrone, C. 1952. Certain aspects of gynecologic practice in the late nineteenth century. *Am. J. Surgery* 84: 95–106.

Ulfelder, H. 1979. The current status of stilbestrol disorders. *Surgical Rounds,* January, pp. 50–53.

———. 1980. The stilbestrol disorders in historical perspective. *Cancer* 45: 3008–3011.

United States Department of Health, Education and Welfare. 1978. *Information for physicians: DES exposure In Utero.* DHEW Publication no. (NIH) 78–1119.

United States Department of Health and Human Services, Centers for Disease Control (Atlanta, Ga. 30333). *Morbidity and Mortality Weekly,* 24 April 1981. (Summary of epidemiologic and demographic features of women aged 15–44 having hysterectomies in the United States.)

Veith, I. 1965. *Hysteria: The history of a disease.* Chicago: University of Chicago Press.

Veridiano, N. P., Delke, I., Rogers, J., and Tancer, M. L. 1980. Reproductive performance of DES-exposed female progeny. *Ob. Gyn.* 58: 58–61.

Veridiano, N. P., Tancer, M. L., and Weiner, E. A. 1978. Squamous cell carcinoma *in situ* of the vagina and cervix after intrauterine DES exposure. *Ob. Gyn.* 52 (suppl.): 30–33.

Vessey, M. P., Fairweather, D. V. J., Norman-Smith, R., and Buckley, J. 1983. A randomized double-blind controlled trial of the value of stilboestrol therapy in pregnancy: Long-term follow-up of mothers and their offspring. *Brit. J. Ob. Gyn.* 90: 1007–1017.

Vital and Health Statistics. 1977. Characteristics of visits to female and male physicians (data from the National Ambulatory Medical Care Survey, U.S., series 13, no. 49). DHHS Publication no. (PHS) 80-1710.

Vooijs, P. G., Ng, A. B., and Wentz, W. B. 1973. The detection of vaginal adenosis and clear-cell carcinoma. *Acta Cytol.* 17: 59–63.

Wade, N. 1972. DES: A case study of regulatory abdication. *Science* 177: 335–37.

Walker, J., MacGillivray, I., Macnaughton, M. C. 1976. *Combined textbook of obstetrics and gynecology.* 9th ed. Edinburgh: Churchill Livingstone.

Warnes, H. 1972. The traumatic syndrome. *Can. Psych. Assoc. J.* 17: 391–96.

Washington Post. 1981. Univ. Md. doctor gives DES to retarded youths. 15 November.

Weigert, E. 1970. The cult and mythology of the Magna Mater from the standpoint of psychoanalysis. In *The courage to love: Selected papers of Edith Weigert,* pp. 299–357. New Haven: Yale University Press.

Weinstein, M. C. 1980. Estrogen use in postmenopausal women: Costs, risks and benefits. *New Eng. J. Med.* 303: 308–15.

Weiss, N. P. 1977. Mother, the invention of necessity: Dr. Benjamin Spock's *Baby and child care. American Q.* 29: 519–46.

Wells, T. S., Hegar, A., and Battey, R. 1886. Castration in mental and nervous diseases: A symposium. *Am. J. Med. Sci.* 92: 455–90.

Werner, A., and Schneider, J. M. 1974. Teaching medical students interactional skills: A research-based course in the doctor-patient relationship. *New Eng. J. Med.* 290: 1232–1237.

White, P., and Hunt, H. 1940. Prediction and prevention of pregnancy accidents in diabetes. *JAMA* 115: 2039–2040.

———. 1943. Pregnancy complicating diabetes: A report of clinical results. *J. Clin. Endocrinology* 3: 500–11.

White, P., Koshy, P., and Duckers, J. 1953. The management of pregnancy complicating diabetes and of children of diabetic mothers. *Med. Clin. N. Amer.* 37: 1481–1496.

Whitehead, A. N. 1933. *Adventures of ideas.* Chap. 6, pp. 110–26. New York: Macmillan.

Whitehead, M. I., Townsend, P. T., Pryse-Davies, J., Ryder, T. A., and King, R. J. B. 1981. Effects of estrogens and progestins on the biochemistry and morphology of the postmenopausal endometrium. *New Eng. J. Med.* 305: 1599–1605.

Wilkins, R. T., and Sandifer, S. H. 1979. Follow-up on the problem of increased incidence of thyroid carcinoma from the effects of childhood irradiation. *J. Family Practice* 8: 265–72.

Wilson, J. D., George, F. W., and Griffin, J. E. 1981. The hormonal control of sexual development. In Naftolin and Butz 1981, pp. 1278–1284.

Wilson, R. A., Brevetti, R. E., and Wilson, T. A. 1963. Specific procedures for the elimination of the menopause. *Western J. Surg. Ob. Gyn.* 71: 110–21.

Wilson, R. A., and Wilson, T. A. 1963. The fate of the nontreated postmenopausal woman: A plea for the maintenance of adequate estrogen from puberty to the grave. *J. Am. Geriatrics Soc.* 11:347–62.

Winston, M., Winston, S., Appelbaum, P. S., and Rhoden, N. K. 1982. Case studies: Can a subject consent to a "Ulysses Contract"? *Hastings Center Report* 12, August.

Wolfe, S. M. 1978. Evidence of breast cancer from DES and current precribing of DES and other estrogens. Statement to the Obstetrics and Gynecology Advisory Committee of the FDA, 30 January.

Women and Health Roundtable, vol. 5, no. 10. 1981. Complete issue on DES.

Wood, A. D. 1973. The fashionable diseases: Women's complaints and their treatment in nineteenth century America. *J. Interdisc. Hist.* 4: 25–52.

Yalom, I. D., Green, R., and Fisk, N. 1973. Prenatal exposure to female hormones: Effect on psychosexual development in boys. *Arch. Gen. Psychiatry.* 28: 554–61.

Yesavage, J. A. 1983. Dangerous behavior by Vietnam veterans with schizophrenia. *Am. J. Psychiatry* 140: 1180–1183.

Young, J. H. 1967. *The medical messiahs: A social history of health quackery in twentieth century America.* Princeton: Princeton University Press.

Youngs, D. D., and Ehrhardt, A. A. 1980. *Psychosomatic obstetrics and gynecology.* New York: Appleton Century Crofts.

Zinberg, N. E., ed. 1964. Psychiatry and medical practice in a general hospital. New York: International Universities Press.

Zola, I. K. 1972. Medicine as an institution of social control. *Soc. Rev.* 20: 487–504. Also in *The Cultural Crisis of Modern Medicine,* John Ehrenreich, ed. 1978. New York: Monthly Review Press.

Zondek, B., and Aschheim, S. 1927. Hypophysenrorderlappen und ovarium: Beziehungen der endokrinen Drüsen zur Ovarialfunktion. *Arch. f. Gynak.* 130: a.

Zugaib, M. 1982. Efeitos da administracao de estrogênios sobe a hemodinâmica uterina ea producao de progesterona em ovelhas gravidas. Ph.D. diss., Sao Paulo (in Portuguese).

Zuspan, F. P., and Christian, C. D. 1983. *Reids' controversy in obstetrics and gynecology.* Vol. 3. Philadelphia: Saunders.

Index